PERMANENT WEIGHT LOSS

THE NO NONSENSE LIBRARY

NO NONSENSE HEALTH GUIDES

Women's Health and Fitness
A Diet for Lifetime Health
A Guide to Exercise and Fitness Equipment
How to Tone and Trim Your Trouble Spots
Stretch for Health
Unstress Your Life
Calories, Carbohydrates and Sodium
All about Vitamins and Minerals
Your Emotional Health and Well-Being
Reducing Cholesterol

OTHER NO NONSENSE GUIDES

CAR GUIDES

CAREER GUIDES

COOKING GUIDES

FINANCIAL GUIDES

LEGAL GUIDES

PARENTING GUIDES

PHOTOGRAPHY GUIDES

REAL ESTATE GUIDES

STUDY GUIDES

SUCCESS GUIDES

WINE GUIDES

NO NONSENSE HEALTH GUIDE®

PERMANENT WEIGHT LOSS

An Easy, Sensible Program for a Slimmer You

By the Editors of
PREVENTION® Magazine

Longmeadow Press

Notice

This book is intended as a reference volume only, not as a medical manual or guide to self-treatment. It is not intended as a substitute for the medical advice of physicians. The reader should regularly consult a physician in general, and particularly for any symptoms. If you suspect that you have a medical problem, we urge you to seek competent medical help. Keep in mind that exercise and nutritional needs vary from person to person, depending on age, sex, health status and individual variations. The information here is intended to help you make informed decisions about your health, not as a substitute for any treatment that may have been prescribed by your doctor.

Library of Congress Cataloging-in-Publication Data

Permanent weight loss.

    (No nonsense health guide)
    1. Low-calorie diet.
I. Prevention (Emmaus, Pa.)   II. Series: No nonsense health guide.
RM222.2.P4345   1989   613.2'5   88-26862
ISBN 0-681-40716-6 paperback

Compiled and edited by Marcia Holman and Jane Sherman

Book design by Acey Lee
Cover illustration by Jean Gardner

Photographs by Christopher Barone p. 38; Julian Baum p. 3; Angelo M. Caggiano p. 45; David Keith p. 4; Alison Miksch p. 23; Rodale Press Photography Department pp. 51, 80; Christie C. Tito p. 31.

Printed in the United States of America

0 9 8 7 6 5 4 3 2

Contents

Introduction: Winning the Weight-Loss War vii

Chapter 1: The Experts' Guide to Successful Weight Loss 1
The best ways to lose pounds permanently, from the Health,
Weight and Stress Clinic of Johns Hopkins Medical
Institution.

Chapter 2: Is Your Diet Draining Away Nutrients? 21
Your diet may make vitamins and minerals vanish along
with the pounds. You're better off counting nutrients, not
calories.

Chapter 3: Think Yourself Slim 28
The key to successful weight loss is partly psychological.
Learn to develop a positive self-image.

Chapter 4: Help Your Body Melt Fat 35
How to get your metabolism moving so calories burn faster.

Chapter 5: Get Your Mate to Help You Lose Weight 40
A supportive partner can make dieting easier. Here's how
to turn a dieting foe into a helpful friend.

Chapter 6: Sip Your Way to Slimness 46
A guide to leaner liquids that quench thirst without quan-
tities of calories.

Chapter 7: Eat Out and Lose Weight 58
It's possible to dine out without piling on the pounds. Here's
how to order foods that are flavorful without adding fat.

Chapter 8: The Best Ways to Flatten Your Belly 65
There are right ways and wrong ways to tone your tummy.
Leading fitness experts help you tell the difference.

Chapter 9: How to Improve the Rotation Diet 69
The weak points in the popular reducing plan can be
overcome, experts say, with these changes.

Chapter 10: 29 Little Ways to Lose a Lot of Weight 77
Pick a bunch of these ideas and see how quickly losing
weight stops being a losing battle.

Chapter 11: Fat-Removal Surgery: The Inside Story. 81
Is it safe to have your fat suctioned, your stomach stapled?
Do these operations really work? Here's what you need to
know before undergoing surgery to slice away unsightly
pounds.

Winning the Weight-Loss War

Everywhere you look today, there is evidence of the ongoing "battle of the bulge" being waged by many Americans. You can see it in the proliferation of health spas and racquetball clubs, in the increasing numbers of walkers and runners, in the seemingly endless succession of diet books and "workout" videotapes, in fast-food restaurants that feature salad bars and in supermarkets amply stocked with low-calorie this and low-fat that.

Make no mistake: This is no mere fad, for Americans are indeed bulging. A National Health and Nutrition Examination survey conducted several years ago determined that 32 percent of adult men and 36 percent of adult women were 10 percent or more above average weight. Nor has the situation improved: Indications are that the incidence of overweight is still rising. By any standard measure, obesity is commonplace in the United States.

Given these facts, it's hard to believe that throughout most of history, one of life's most difficult tasks actually has been getting enough food to survive. In the United States and other Western societies, however, modern agricultural techniques and technological advances have produced a cornucopia of palatable foods. With so much temptation so readily available, overweight may be a natural—though not inevitable—consequence.

Most of us who *are* overweight don't need anyone to tell us about it. All we need to do is look in the mirror. What people want to know is, what can be done about it? In short, can we win the battle of the bulge?

The answer is simple—yes. Most people *can* lose weight or prevent weight gain, experts insist. That's what *Permanent Weight Loss* is all about. It's not a diet book and it's not an exercise book, although you'll learn about diet and exercise. It's a book about weight loss—how to lose weight and, more important, how to keep it off. Whether you want to launch a major weight-loss effort or whittle off those last five or ten stubborn pounds, this book shows you that it's just as easy to slim down and stay that way. No gimmicks, no gadgets, no forbidden foods—just a sensible guide to slimming successfully by changing everyday habits.

The Experts' Guide to Successful Weight Loss

Maria Simonson, Ph.D., Sc.D., took the "practice what you preach" dictum a step further. She preaches what she practiced.

Seventeen years ago, the founder and director of the Health, Weight and Stress Clinic weighed 345 pounds—the result of months and months of self-pity eating as she recovered from a stroke.

Then she and 15 overweight co-workers at the Johns Hopkins University School of Hygiene decided to form a self-help group. After trying—and failing—with a number of commercial weight-loss groups, they struck out on their own, tapping into the vast resources of the Johns Hopkins University Medical institutions and Hospital.

All of the group lost weight—Dr. Simonson is now half her previous size—and their success attracted the attention of Hopkins physicians, who asked if their overweight patients might join. The Health, Weight and Stress Clinic was born.

Over 40,000 people have achieved success in the program. Dr. Simonson, now professor emeritus at Johns Hopkins, has even taken it to the skies. She's a consultant and medical research director for the International Flight Attendants Association, which draws from 33 major U.S. and foreign airlines.

The diet and weight-loss tips in this chapter are the direct result of nearly 20 years of her experience and that of her staff—many of whom are professionals who volunteer—and ex-patients. They learned that losing weight and keeping it off isn't simply a matter of eating less and exercising more but of understanding the particular physical, psychological, nutritional and environmental factors that make us overeat in the first place.

Most important, says Dr. Simonson, is to remember, "Weight loss is not success. It's an achievement. To maintain that loss for 18 months to two years within five pounds is success."

It's also a lot of work—and the best time to start is now.

If you need any further motivation, take a look at the photos on the next two pages for examples of the positive results that can come from the weight-loss methods described in this chapter.

Do You Know Your Type?

If you try to lose weight without knowing what caused you to gain weight in the first place, you may simply be inviting failure. You may lose 1 pound or 100, but if you don't get to the root of your problem, you're likely to see those pounds piling back on. According to Dr. Simonson's theory, "We can correct bad habits by finding out why we do them."

Take a look at this list of physical and psychological types of overeaters, developed in large part by Frank Bigsby, M.D., of Tulane University. You may find that one best describes you—or that up to three explain your overweight. Though some detail genetic or physical characteristics that contribute to obesity, the majority are psychological characteristics. Surveys show that 85 percent of all overweight people use eating to solve their emotional problems.

We've included some special tips with a few of these psychological profiles, but the suggestions in the section, 50 Top Diet Tips, which follows, should help you no matter which type of eater you are. Actually, once you know your type, you're on your way to the self-awareness that will help you win the fight against fat.

Familial or constitutional obesity.   Your whole family is overweight. You eat large, farm-family meals. The whole family

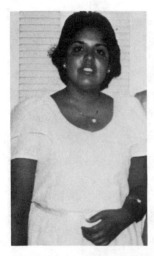

BETTY BACA
Pounds lost: 60
Weight-loss method:
  Ate mostly chicken, fish, fruit
  and vegetables
Type of exercise used:
  Running, weight training
Length of time to goal:
  2 years

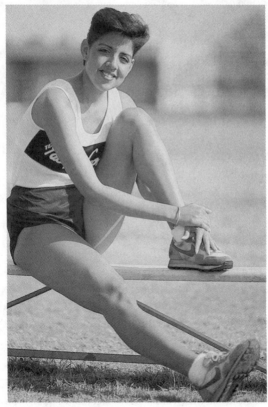

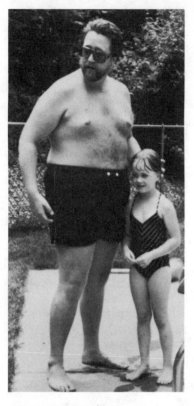 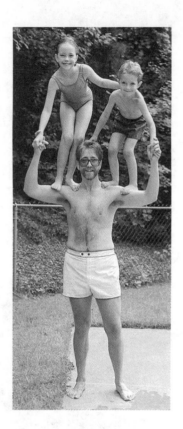

BILL ANDERSON
Pounds lost: 140
Weight-loss method: Behavior modification, life-style change
Type of exercise used: Swimming, walking
Length of time to goal: 18 months

may even snack together in front of the television at night. You probably love to cook and are sedentary. (This is not necessarily a genetic problem but one of faulty nutrition.) *Special tip:* You and your family need nutritional counseling and may need psychotherapy if there is a family problem contributing to your obesity.

The habit eater.   You were larger than most of your class-mates as a child. You have a big body, with pronounced muscular and skeletal development. You don't skip meals—in fact, you may eat balanced, nutritional meals—but your diet may contain a lot of starches. You're a time-clock eater, always having lunch at noon whether you're hungry or not. *Special tip:* You need motivation. Try Diet Tip 8 later in this chapter.

Pubertal obesity.   You are a teen who matured sexually before most of your classmates. As you grew, you found your appetite had grown as well, and you developed cravings for sweets. You may be active, but not necessarily. Your motivation to lose weight may only come when you notice the opposite sex—and notice they're noticing you. *Special tip:* You usually have, and need, strong parental support to keep you on a diet. Don't try to give up all your favorite foods at once. Learn to control portions instead.

Gastronomic obesity.   You are probably a man or woman who loves to cook. You're not interested in quantity as much as quality. You'd call yourself a gourmet. You're probably not seriously overweight. In fact, you may have only noticed those few extra pounds when you hit your thirties and forties. You're not an emotional eater, nor do you snack, which works in your favor. *Special tip:* You can benefit by group support (see Diet Tip 8 in the following section) and by learning portion control, so you eat the same good food but less of it. You can also benefit from Diet Tip 25.

The night eater.   You're virtuous all day, but at nightfall the nonstop snacking begins. You may have insomnia or be a habitual coffee drinker or smoker. You may fall into one of three different classes of night eater. There's the after-dinner eater who may have skipped meals during the day. There's the late-late-night eater who wakes up and builds and devours a Dagwood sandwich as a snack before he's able to fall back to sleep. The late-late-night eater may be responding to the true physiological hunger caused by a drop in blood sugar or cerebral ischemia, a restricted flow of blood to the brain. For this person, a prebed snack or a few slices of orange at bedside can help. There's also the night owl, whose circadian rhythms make him hungry every few hours or so. *Special tip:* See Diet Tips 1, 9 and 11 later in this chapter.

The compulsive eater.   You're a nutritional garbage disposal. Your emotional state is unstable and you are probably very overweight.

You can nibble all day long, may always be cooking and will eat food off other people's plates. Sweets and starches are your favorite snacks, and you aren't above sneaking and hiding food. Food is your emotional comfort or a weapon. *Special tip:* Consider counseling or therapy.

The excessive liquid drinker.   The coffee pot is always on at your house. You're rarely seen without a cup or glass of something in your hand. You're very much like the compulsive eater, only it's something to drink—not a snack. You're under a lot of stress and may drink a lot of liquids instead of eating, which seriously compromises your nutrition. You can drink up to 20 diet sodas a day, which, because they're high in sodium, cause you to retain water and leaves you bloated and feeling overweight even if you're not.

The pregnant father.   Your wife is pregnant, but you're the one who's gaining weight. You may not feel ready to have this baby. You feel rejected, insecure, even jealous. You may be eating as a substitute for sex. *Special tip:* Family counseling may be of some help.

The "fat phobic" or "former fatty."   You're likely a woman, not overweight now but probably overweight as a teen and deathly afraid to gain weight. Obsessed by your weight, you are probably rather thin. You aren't anorectic, but you eat very low-calorie meals or crash diet. You may insist that family members also share your obsession. Despite that, your children may be compulsive overeaters, mostly in rebellion. *Special tip:* Family counseling is recommended.

Disability obesity.   You broke your leg skiing or you had your gallbladder removed and have been bedridden for weeks. Perhaps you had a stroke. Chances are, your inactivity is putting the weight on. But you may be using your illness or disability as an excuse to deny reality: "I can eat what I want and won't gain an ounce because I'm sick." *Special tip:* Physical therapy may help.

Sedentary obesity.   You probably dreaded gym class as a child. Today, you still avoid physical activity, largely because you're so overweight. If you're older and your metabolism has slowed down, you may be gaining weight at an even more rapid rate. You're under a great deal of stress and may be very frustrated.

The chronic dieter.   You know the calorie count of everything you eat and have been on every diet known to mankind, but you still can't lose weight. You want immediate and rapid weight loss—fad diets and weight-loss gimmicks are designed for you—and you think you know more than the experts, despite your chronic failure to solve your weight problem. *Special tip:* You need special motivation. Try preparing your favorite meal and sitting down to eat it naked in front of a mirror. Suitably horrified, take a no nonsense approach to the diet.

The environmental and occupational overeater. You're an extrovert who frequently eats lunch or dinner out, entertaining clients or traveling for business. You may be a shift worker whose meal schedule is out of kilter with the rest of the world, or a high school student working in a fast-food restaurant or ice-cream shop, where fattening foods are the only game in town.

Middle-age obesity.   It can start as early as your thirties. Your metabolic rate slows and you're no longer burning calories as efficiently. Instead, you're storing them as fat. You may have been thin or slightly plump all your life until you suddenly started gaining. You may have dental problems that make it difficult to eat anything but creamy, fattening foods. You may have less money and can't afford nutritious foods, or you're doing fine and all the dining out and cruises are putting on the pounds.

Adolescent or developmental obesity.   You're a teenager who is tense, a compulsive snacker and quite overweight. You find it difficult to tolerate frustration or delay gratification. You are withdrawn, unsociable and may have family problems. Food is a common cause of fights in your home. *Special tip:* You and your parents probably need psychological and nutritional counseling.

Nutritional obesity.   You're not seriously overweight, but your knowledge of nutrition is nil. Your total caloric intake isn't excessive, but your diet is notoriously out of balance. You may experience the 4:00 P.M. slump and may drink a lot of black coffee. *Special tip:* You need the guidance of a nutritionist to help you eat better-balanced meals.

Climacteric obesity.   You're a menopausal woman or have recently had a hysterectomy. The hormonal disturbance not only adds to your weight problem but aggravates emotional problems as well. *Special tip:* Have a thorough physical to determine if you have a hormone imbalance. Also consider counseling to help you adjust.

Extreme obesity.   You may weigh 200 to 300 pounds or more and may be constitutionally big at the same time. Your diet lacks balance and you may drink a lot of coffee. *Special tip:* You should see your physician before undertaking any diet program.

50 Top Diet Tips

These diet ideas come from the staff and patients at the Johns Hopkins Health, Weight and Stress Clinic.

1. Start your diet with a food diary. Record what you eat, what you were doing at the time, how you felt. That tells you about yourself—your temptation times, the emotional states that encourage you to nosh—and may help you lose once you see how much you eat.
2. Bill Heidel's Law: When tempted, ask yourself, Do I really want to eat that or do I want to be thin? (Bill Heidel went from 535 pounds to 165 pounds in two years on the program.)
3. If you're about to cheat, allow yourself a treat, then eat only half and throw the other half away.
4. When hunger hits, wait ten minutes before eating and see if it passes.
5. Instead of eating the forbidden piece of candy, brush your teeth. The fresh, sweet taste of the toothpaste may take your craving away.
6. Set attainable goals. Don't say, "I want to lose 150 pounds." Say, "I want to lose 5 pounds this month."
7. Drink six to eight glasses of water a day. Water itself helps cut down on water retention because it acts as a diuretic. Taken before meals, it dulls the appetite by giving you that full feeling.
8. Diet with a buddy. The program at Johns Hopkins relies heavily on support groups: caring people who help one another succeed. Start your own, even with just one other person.

9. Avoid evening TV. Studies show people who watch a lot of TV tend to be overweight. Overweight people will tell you that TV encourages them not only to sit still but to snack.

10. Substitute activity for eating. When the cravings hit, go to the health club, or dust, or walk around the block. This is especially helpful if you eat out of anger.

11. If you're a late-late-night eater, have a carbohydrate, such as a slice of bread or a cracker, before bedtime to cut down on cravings. Keep an orange slice or a glass of water by your bed to quiet the hunger pangs that wake you up.

12. Go ahead and buy the candy, but don't eat it right away. If you wait, you might decide it's not worth the calories.

13. If you use food as a reward, establish a new reward system. Buy yourself flowers instead of candy.

14. In your food diary, write down everything you eat—everything, including what you taste when you cook. If you monitor what you eat, you can't go off the diet.

15. If you plateau at a certain weight, don't panic. It's your body getting used to the new you. Drink water, increase your exercise or reduce your calories (don't go below 1,000) to give you the boost you need.

16. Weigh yourself once a week at the same time. Your weight fluctuates constantly, and you can weigh more at night than you did in the morning, a downer if you stuck to your diet all day.

17. Feel like you're about to really pig out? Quickly suck on something sour—a pickle or a lemon. If you suck it for a while, you may eliminate your cravings.

18. If you want something sweet, eat the smallest amount of fruit or sip the tiniest amount of fruit juice you can to get you through the crisis.

19. If the pie on the counter is just too great a temptation and you don't want to throw it away, freeze it.

20. Make your own sweet drink by adding a little bit of vanilla to ice water with some artificial sweetener.

21. If a binge is about to strike, do your nails. A couple of coats of polish take some time to dry, and by then the danger could pass.

The Weather Made Me Eat It

If you're having trouble figuring out why on certain days you're more likely to pig out, keep track of the weather in your food diary. Maria Simonson, Ph.D., Sc.D., has discovered that wind, temperature and precipitation can all have an effect on mood and appetite.

Hot weather usually dulls your desire for food, but the first chill could send you to the grocery store. Rain makes some people depressed, and if they're prone, they can turn to food for comfort. Winds like the Santa Anas in California can make you hungry. Sometimes, when barometric pressure drops, you can swell up as much as an inch a day, says Dr. Simonson. Women between 35 and 50 tend to be more weather sensitive than other people.

So if you've put on weight and you know you didn't cheat, or you're hungry for no good reason, check in with your local meteorologist.

22. Eat foods from gray, green or brown plates. Studies show these colors make you eat less. Blue and green stimulate the eye less than orange and yellow.

23. Use visualization. Imagine yourself ten pounds heavier. Then add a few more pounds. Ask yourself if you still really want to eat. Then close your eyes and imagine yourself at your ideal weight.

24. Forget the ugly-picture-on-the-refrigerator trick. It will just make you depressed. Place a picture of yourself at your thinnest—or one of your favorite celebrity whose shape you admire—to give you something real to work toward.

25. Make dining an event. Eat from your own special plate, on your own special placemat, and borrow the Japanese art of arranging food to make your meal, however meager, look lovely. This is a trick that helps chronic overeaters and bingers

pay attention to their food instead of consuming it unconsciously.

26. Don't shop when you're hungry. You'll only buy more fattening food.

27. Avoid finger foods that are easy to eat in large amounts.

28. Avoid consuming large quantities of fattening liquids, which are so easy to overdo. That includes alcohol.

29. Keep plenty of crunchy foods like raw veggies and air-popped popcorn on hand. They're high in fiber, satisfying and filling.

30. Always leave something on your plate, even if you're a charter member of the Clean Plate Club. It's a good sign that you can stop eating when you want to, not just when your plate is empty.

31. Eat with a cocktail fork.

32. Don't deprive yourself. Eating too few calories or abandoning your favorite foods will make you feel terrible and may drive you back to your overeating habits. Have ice cream, but just a little. And be happy with a slower weight loss. Remember, you're less likely to gain back what you lose slowly, and your body isn't going to sag.

33. Always eat at the table, never in front of the TV set or with the radio on. Concentrate on eating every mouthful slowly and savoring each morsel.

34. Use chopsticks. Unless you're really adept, you'll be forced to eat slower and take smaller bites.

35. Always eat with a utensil—even finger foods like fruit or bread.

36. Chew everything from 10 to 20 times—and count.

37. Wear a belt or girdle that makes you aware when you've eaten enough.

38. When eating out, eat your salad first, with low-calorie dressing or lemon, to dull your appetite before the entrée.

39. Lose weight for yourself—not your husband, your mother or your friends.

40. Recognize the times you're most vulnerable to snacking (make special note in your food diary) and make sure you have either low-calorie snacks handy for those times, or get thoroughly occupied with something constructive or fun.

41. Make the kitchen off-limits at any time other than mealtime.
42. If your usual route takes you too close to a tempting sweet shop or by a hot dog vendor, blaze some new, nonfattening trails.
43. Use smaller plates than usual.
44. Never skip meals, especially breakfast. Schedule all your meals and snacks at regular intervals so you don't get hungry between.
45. Get enough sleep—but not too much.
46. Try to avoid sugar; it tends to make you crave more and more.
47. Lose two more pounds than your ideal weight to give you some leeway when your weight fluctuates.
48. To maintain your weight, add 350 to 500 calories a day to your diet, but do it gradually—about 100 calories at a time—so you know when maintenance stops and gaining begins.
49. Plan ahead. Know what you're going to have to eat tomorrow and schedule leftovers into your meal plans. A weekly meal planner is ideal.
50. Avoid late-night meals. That's when your metabolism is less likely to burn up those calories. Studies have shown that people who eat 2,000 calories in the morning lose more weight than those who eat the same amount at night.

No More Calorie Counting

The diets on the following pages, which were designed by Johns Hopkins University nutritionists, are based on a food-exchange list similar to that prescribed for diabetics. Choose from the 1,000-, 1,200-, or 1,500- or 1,800-calorie diets. To help you decide which is best for you, find out how many calories you are now consuming daily and subtract 500 to 1,000.

The 1,000-calorie diet is meant only for starters. It should help you drop quite a few pounds quickly— that's for morale purposes—but you should stay on it only for one to two weeks. It's not safe to stay on it longer.

Each of the diets has been developed so that you don't have to count calories. They're already counted for you, as long as you adhere strictly to the number of exchanges and serving sizes of each food. You can eat only the allotted number of exchanges for each food group. For instance, in the 1,200-calorie diet, you're permitted two milk exchanges, which means, for example, you can have two cups of skim milk a day, or two cups of unflavored yogurt and so on. You will note, however, that some of the milk exchanges—whole milk, for instance—are also marked as fat exchanges. That's because they contain substantial amounts of fat. Take that into account when you're planning your fat exchanges every day.

You also can't interchange foods from different lists. If you don't like milk, you can't substitute apple juice or orange juice from the fruit lists. They're not equivalent nutritionally or calorically.

Though most of the exchange lists are self-explanatory, please take special note of the meat and fish exchanges. Many of the exchanges are only one ounce of meat or fish. On the 1,200-calorie diet, you're allowed five meat or fish exchanges. You can choose to have them all at one meal—five ounces of white-

(continued)

No More Calorie Counting —
Continued

meat chicken with all the fat removed, for example — or spread over the day: an egg in the morning, two ounces of chicken in a sandwich at lunch and two ounces of shrimp for dinner.

Your fruit exchanges work in the same way. You can choose three fruits of the appropriate size (a quarter of a cantaloupe, one small nectarine and a medium peach) or one larger piece of fruit (three-quarters of a cantaloupe) or have some fruit and some juice.

Once you start, you should find the going easy and simple. In fact, here's a sample 1,200-calorie menu to let you know what you're in for. Check it against the diet and exchange lists so you can see how it's done.

Sample Menu

Breakfast

    1 fruit: ¼ cantaloupe
    1 meat/fish: 1 boiled egg
    1 bread: 1 slice toast
    1 fat: 1 teaspoon margarine
    1 milk: 1 cup skim milk
    Coffee or tea

Lunch

    2 meat/fish: 2 ounces sliced chicken
    2 bread: 2 slices whole wheat toast
    1 fat: 1 teaspoon mayonnaise
    1 vegetable: Lettuce and tomato (up to ½ cup tomato)
    1 fruit: 1 pear
    1 milk: 1 cup skim milk

Dinner

    2 meat/fish: 2 ounces broiled flounder with lemon
    1 bread: 1 small baked potato

1 fat: 1 tablespoon sour cream
2 vegetable: 1 cup broccoli
1 bread: 1 roll
1 fruit: ¾ cup strawberries
Coffee, tea or other noncaloric drink

Choose Your Diet

1,000-Calorie Diet Daily Exchange Units

Milk: 2 exchanges
Vegetable: 2 exchanges
Fruit: 3 exchanges
Bread, cereal, cracker, starchy vegetable: 3 exchanges
Meat or fish: 5 exchanges
Fat: 2 exchanges

1,200-Calorie Diet Daily Exchange Units

Milk: 2 exchanges
Vegetable: 3 exchanges
Fruit: 3 exchanges
Bread, cereal, cracker, starchy vegetable: 5 exchanges
Meat or fish: 5 exchanges
Fat: 2 exchanges

1,500-Calorie Diet Daily Exchange Units

Milk: 2 exchanges
Vegetable: 2 exchanges
Fruit: 5 exchanges
Bread, cereal, cracker, starchy vegetable: 7 exchanges
Meat or fish: 6 exchanges
Fat: 4 exchanges

1,800-Calorie Diet Daily Exchange Units

Milk: 2 exchanges
Vegetable: 4 exchanges

(continued)

No More Calorie Counting —
Continued

Fruit: 5 exchanges
Bread, cereal, cracker, starchy vegetable: 7 exchanges
Meat or fish: 7 exchanges
Fat: 4 exchanges

Exchange Lists

Milk Exchanges (80 calories)

  1 cup skim, nonfat milk
  1 cup 1% fat fortified milk (½ fat*)
  1 cup 2% fat fortified milk (1 fat*)
  1 cup whole milk (2 fat*)
  1 cup plain skim-milk yogurt
  1 cup plain yogurt from 2% fat fortified milk (1 fat*)
  ⅓ cup powdered milk (measured without liquid)
  1 cup plain yogurt from whole milk (2 fat*)
  ½ cup canned evaporated skim milk
  ½ cup canned evaporated whole milk (2 fat*)
  1 cup buttermilk from skim milk
  1 cup buttermilk from whole milk (2 fat*)

Vegetable Exchanges (½-cup portions, 25 calories)

Asparagus, bean sprouts, beets, broccoli, brussels sprouts, cabbage, carrots, cauliflower, celery, eggplant, green peppers, mushrooms, okra, onions, rhubarb, rutabaga, salad greens (beet, chard, collards, dandelion, kale, mustard, spinach, turnip), sauerkraut, string beans (green/yellow), summer squash, tomatoes, tomato juice, turnips, vegetable juice, zucchini

Free Vegetables (these vegetables can be eaten as frequently as desired)

Chicory, Chinese cabbage, cucumbers, endive, escarole, lettuce, parsley, radishes, watercress

*Counts as specified fat exchange.

Fruit Exchanges

  1 small apple
  ⅓ cup apple juice (unsweetened)
  ½ cup applesauce (unsweetened)
  2 medium apricots (fresh)
  4 halves apricots (dried)
  ½ small banana
  ½ cup blackberries
  ½ cup blueberries
  ½ cup raspberries
  ¾ cup strawberries
 10 large cherries
  ⅓ cup cider
  ¾ cup cranberry juice[†]
  2 dates
  1 fig (fresh)
  1 fig (dried)
  ½ cup fruit cocktail
  ½ cup grapefruit
  ½ cup grapefruit juice (unsweetened)
 12 grapes
  ½ small mango
  ¼ small cantaloupe
  ⅛ medium honeydew
  1 cup watermelon
  1 small nectarine
  1 small orange
  ½ cup orange juice (unsweetened)
  ¾ cup papaya
  1 medium peach
  1 small pear

[†]Cranberries may be used as desired if no sugar is added.

(continued)

No More Calorie Counting —
Continued

1 medium persimmon
2 slices or 1 cup pineapple
⅓ cup pineapple juice (unsweetened)
2 medium plums
2 medium prunes
¼ cup prune juice (unsweetened)
2 tablespoons raisins
1 medium tangerine

Bread, Cereal, Cracker, Starchy Vegetable Exchanges (68 calories each)

Breads

1 slice white, whole wheat or rye
½ small whole wheat bagel
½ whole wheat English muffin
1 plain roll, bread
½ hamburger or hot dog bun
3 tablespoons dried bread crumbs
1 tortilla (6-inch)

Cereals

⅓ cup All-Bran or Bran Buds
½ cup bran flakes
¾ cup cornflakes
1 Shredded Wheat biscuit
¼ cup Grape-Nuts
¾ cup other ready-to-eat cereal
1 cup puffed cereal (unfrosted)
½ cup cooked cereal or grits
½ cup rice or barley (cooked)
½ cup pasta
2 cups popcorn (no fat)

2 tablespoons cornmeal (dry)
2½ tablespoons rye or whole wheat flour
¼ cup wheat germ

Crackers

3 arrowroot
2 graham (2½-inch square)
½ matzoh (4 × 6-inch)
5 slices melba toast
20 oyster crackers
25 pretzels (3⅛ × ⅛-inch)
3 rye wafers (2 × 3½-inch)
6 saltines
4 soda (2½-inch square)

Starchy vegetables

⅓ cup corn
1 small corn on the cob
½ cup dried beans or peas (cooked)
½ cup lima beans
⅔ cup parsnips
½ cup green peas
½ cup potato (mashed)
1 small white potato (baked)
¾ cup pumpkin
½ cup winter squash
¼ cup yam or sweet potato

Meat Exchanges (55 calories)

1 ounce lean meat, fish or poultry
1 ounce skim-milk cheese
1 hot dog (average)
1 egg

(continued)

No More Calorie Counting—
Continued

¼ cup low-cholesterol egg substitute

5 clams, oysters, medium shrimp

¼ cup crabmeat or lobster

1 ounce salmon or tuna (water-packed)

1 ounce medium sardines (drained)

¼ cup cottage cheese (1% fat)

Fat Exchanges (45 calories)

⅛ avocado (4-inch)

1 slice bacon (cooked crisp)

1 teaspoon butter

1 teaspoon margarine

1 teaspoon mayonnaise

2 teaspoons imitation mayonnaise

1 teaspoon salad oil

1 tablespoon French or Italian dressing

2 tablespoons light or sour cream

1 tablespoon cream cheese

2 tablespoons salad dressing

3 tablespoons low-calorie salad dressing

Is Your Diet Draining Away Nutrients?

Too few calories add up to poor nutrition. And poor nutrition can produce poor health.

Hospitals learned that lesson the hard way, says Peter Lindner, M.D., director of continuing medical education for the American Society of Bariatric Physicians (obesity specialists). "That's one of the reasons they added nutritional support services," says Dr. Lindner, who also heads the Lindner Clinic in suburban Los Angeles. "They discovered that some common postoperative infections were not due to the surgery but to poor nutrition."

Researchers have found that immune-system response drops in people on very low-calorie diets, says the physician. "In one study, the researchers were interested in the changes in disease-fighting white blood cells when exposed to vaccine. What they found was that the immune response was reduced in those individuals on improperly administered ultralow-calorie diets, making them more subject to infection. That is probably one of the most dangerous aspects of very low-calorie diets."

If you're a dieter—and surveys show two out of three people are—there's a very good chance you may be endangering your health, warns Dr. Lindner. You may be able to take nutrition for granted when you're eating like a horse, but it becomes critical when you start eating like a bird.

"A good, balanced diet in the higher caloric range probably gives you all the vitamins and minerals you need. It gives you some leeway to play with," says Dr. Lindner. "Drop it down to 800 or 1,000 calories and everything counts."

In fact, according to the Food and Nutrition Board of the National Academy of Sciences—which sets our Recommended Dietary Allowances (RDAs)—it is difficult to get adequate nutrition on diets that provide less than 1,800 to 2,000 calories. Most popular reducing diets call for 1,200 or less.

A Nutritional Balancing Act

It's hard enough to juggle the four food groups into a nutritionally balanced diet when you've got a few thousand calories to work with. Dieters have a tougher task. They have to concoct three healthful meals with roughly half the calories they're used to consuming. And they start out with a handicap—they don't know beans about nutrition.

Following a diet guide may not help. Many popular diet plans are full of dubious nutritional advice. Most dieters know only enough to plan a 1,200-calorie menu down to the last morsel. But knowing calories isn't enough. You can create three low-calorie meals a day without ever straying from the candy counter.

Perhaps the most important thing to remember when you're counting calories is that it's the nutritional value of the calorie that counts. If you don't know the value of a calorie, you don't know what you're missing.

But Paul Lachance, Ph.D., does. Dr. Lachance, professor of nutrition and food science at Rutgers University, evaluated the nutritional content of 11 published weight-loss diets. He chose the 11 because they ran the gamut of popular weight-reducing plans—from high-protein/low-carbohydrate to low-protein/high-carbohydrate, with variations in between. They carried such familiar names as Scarsdale, Stillman, Atkins and the Beverly Hills Diet.

Using the RDAs as a frame of reference, Dr. Lachance and associate dietitian Michele C. Fisher, Ph.D., found that most of the diets were low in thiamine, vitamins B_6 and B_{12}, calcium, iron, zinc and magnesium. Thiamine, vitamins B_6 and B_{12} and magnesium were often at levels of less than 70 percent of the RDA. One, the Beverly Hills Diet, supplied less than 70 percent of the RDAs for more than half of the vitamins and minerals they evaluated, and it was so low in protein that researchers predicted it would lead to a serious protein deficiency over a long period of time.

And there's the rub. Most diets are protracted, if not forever. "Most people stay on a diet for a long time. After all, weight loss doesn't occur overnight," says Dr. Lachance. "If a diet lasts only two weeks, the vitamin and mineral loss is not going to be significant. As far as I'm concerned, women are dieting all the time and may have other risk factors—smoking, contraceptive-pill use—that can affect nutrient metabolism. For them, the loss can be very significant."

In fact, researchers studying otherwise healthy men found that even without those extra risk factors, a prolonged low-calorie diet had a damaging effect on their health. One group, which had previously eaten over 3,000 calories daily, ate about half that for a period of six months. Even though they were eating more calories than prescribed by most reducing diets, the men suffered from depression, anemia,

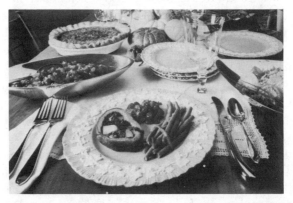

A reducing diet that's too low in calories is likely to shortchange you on nutrition. It's important to eat balanced meals, even if it means adding some calories to your diet plan.

edema, slowing of heartbeat and loss of sex drive. They also tired easily and lacked endurance.

Some weight-loss regimens, specifically those that are mainly protein, can lead to a potentially serious condition called acidosis, which also can occur on fasting diets. In one study, people fed a diet of solely protein and fat lost about two pounds a day—along with large amounts of nitrogen and salt in their urine. They suffered from the symptoms of acidosis, which can include weakness, malaise, headache and heart arrhythmias.

Acidosis can be remedied by adding as little as about three ounces of carbohydrates to the diet.

Needless to say, bizarre diets that rely heavily on one food—such as grapefruit—are going to be nutritionally bankrupt. Very low-calorie liquid diets can be deadly.

Special Advice for Women

Women are always going to have to pay extra attention to the nutrient content of their diets because of their increased needs for certain nutrients. "For women, it's hard enough to get things like calcium and iron," says Cindy Rubin, clinical nutritionist with the obesity research group at the University of Pennsylvania.

Women generally need more iron and calcium than men. "Many women are going to have to supplement their diets with calcium and iron," says noted weight and fitness expert Gabe Mirkin, M.D., who ordinarily doesn't advocate dietary supplements. "One out of four women between 12 and 50 is iron deficient."

Though an iron deficiency may eventually lead to anemia, it has its own immediate health consequences. "When you're iron deficient, even though you're not anemic," says Dr. Mirkin, "you can't clear lactic acid as rapidly as normal from your bloodstream, so you tire earlier at work and play."

"The problem with calcium is that it's scarce except in milk products—the first thing many dieters cut out. Unless you choose skim milk, dairy products can be high in fat and calories," says Dr. Lindner. "It's difficult to get adequate calcium without milk unless you eat sardines, small bones and all."

How food is prepared may also affect a dieter's nutrition. "If you're eating a salad that was tossed three days ago, vitamins are lost simply by exposure," says Dr. Lindner. "If food is cooked too much, you can lose more. Especially at risk are the water-soluble vitamins, such as C and B vitamins."

One of those B vitamins is folate. Women are particularly at risk of developing anemia when they aren't taking in enough folate, which is found in leafy greens. A form of anemia occurs when there isn't enough folate in the body to produce red blood cells. Folate deficiency also has been pinpointed as a factor in a precancerous condition called cervical dysplasia.

Studies have also shown that low-calorie and starvation diets can lead to an excessive loss of zinc, possibly as a result of tissue breakdown. Researchers at the Veterans Administration Hospital in Hines, Illinois, found that weight-loss diets between 600 and 1,240 calories can be zinc deficient, depending on the type and source of dietary protein from which the zinc is derived. Diets that derive most of their protein from red meat tend to supply more zinc that those that rely on chicken, fish, milk products and eggs, which are, unfortunately, the main protein sources of many low-calorie diets.

If it all sounds discouraging, rest assured that the obesity experts understand—and have more than one solution to a dieter's nutritional dilemma.

- If you don't feel you can add red meat to your diet or if time and money constraints make it impossible to eat only freshly prepared foods, you can take supplements. "Theoretically, it's not necessary to supplement your diet," says Dr. Lindner, "but realistically most people don't have the knowledge or the time to do it right. Especially if you're a woman, a standard multiple vitamin that contains iron, B_6, folacin [folate] and zinc along with a calcium supplement should help you make sure you're getting all of the 26 micronutrients you need."
- Learn the value of a calorie. You know there's a big nutritional difference between a 200-calorie candy bar and a 200-calorie protein salad. But even so-called diet foods aren't created equal. "Choose nutrient-dense foods," suggests Cindy Rubin. "For instance, eat broccoli as opposed to lettuce. Both are low in calories, but lettuce is mainly water. You're not getting the heavy doses of vitamin A you get in broccoli."

- Go for variety. Not only is it the spice of life, it improves your chances of getting all the vitamins and minerals you need.
- Plan your diet menu from the four basic food groups. "Each of the major categories represents certain vitamins and minerals," says Dr. Mirkin. "Grains and cereals, for example, give you E and the B vitamins. Fruits and vegetables supply vitamins C and A. If you take in at least 1,500 calories a day and distribute your calories over the four food groups, you'll probably be taking in the nutrients you need."

Eat More and Lose?

The final piece of advice is something of a blockbuster: Eat more calories. By eating more, naturally, you're more likely to meet your nutritional needs. But will you lose weight? Yes, say the experts, as long as you burn up some of those calories through exercise.

In his book *Getting Thin,* Dr. Mirkin advises eating 1,500 calories a day—and using an hour of exercise to burn off 300.

There are some unique advantages to this plan. Aside from losing weight healthfully, you'll stimulate your metabolism to burn even more calories. "You see, diets don't work," says Dr. Mirkin. "When you go on a diet, your metabolism slows down. When you're lying in bed, not even

---

A Word about Exercise

The word is *start.* But start slowly, advises exercise physiologist Rose Dailey. "I encourage our people to do all of the movements they would do naturally. Start with rotating your head while you're still lying in bed, or lifting your chin to your chest. Heavy people shouldn't put stress on their bones, ligaments or tendons. Their range of motion is shortened, so they shouldn't do back bends or high kicks." The best starting-out exercise is walking. "It's aerobic and involves the whole body," says Dailey. Again, start slowly, but work up to three times a week, increasing your distance each time.

moving, you burn 60 calories an hour. If you're on a diet, you burn only 50. If you exercise, you burn 70—without even moving. Exercise speeds up your metabolism 24 hours a day, not to mention suppressing your appetite."

Dr. Mirkin recommends picking two sports—aerobic dancing and biking, for instance—and working up slowly to an hour of each on alternating days. "I specify two sports because it takes you 48 hours to recover, so you should rotate the stressors on your body," he says.

Older people especially need exercise as an integral part of any diet plan. "The two have to be together," says Dr. Lachance. "When you're young, your metabolism is higher and you can get away with more. When you get older, your body changes. Your metabolism slows, your lean body mass goes down and your propensity for adipose [fat] tissue goes up. You lower your need for calories, so if you don't add exercise, you get fat."

Think Yourself Slim

If you have friends who diet all the time but never get slim, ask them how they imagine their lives might be when the years of salads and cravings and premeasured meals are finally over and they attain a stable, comfortable, close-to-ideal weight.

Chances are they will tell you that on such a day their lives will change in so many positive ways. They will be able to wear designer swimwear and fitted shirts. They will be their own best friends. In short, life will be as it should be.

But current wisdom on weight loss—as it applies to those who tend to overeat—is that people are more successful at shedding weight and keeping it off if they start thinking positively about themselves right now, while the pounds are still in place.

Easier said than done, of course. But many psychologists say (and psychology now plays a major role in the weight-loss world) that effective weight loss is easier when people banish negative thought patterns from their minds and replace them with positive ones. Kelly

Brownell, Ph.D., associate professor in the Department of Psychiatry at the University of Pennsylvania School of Medicine and co-director of the Obesity Research Clinic, has studied these negative thoughts. He divides them into four categories.

The first category he calls Dichotomous Thinking. "Overweight people," Dr. Brownell says, "tend to split their lives into two separate compartments. They are either 'on' or 'off' their diets—never in between. We also call this light-bulb thinking, because a light bulb is either on or off.

"For instance, I asked one of the women at the clinic how her diet was going," he says. "She said it was terrible. It turned out that the previous week she had stayed on her 1,200-calorie-a-day diet for six days out of seven. But all she could think about was that she had gone 'off' the diet once. She didn't think positively about the six days she was on it."

He calls the second category of negative thinking The Impossible Dream. Dieters apparently set unrealistic goals for themselves and then feel guilty about not reaching them. "One woman told me that she was going to lose 50 pounds in time for her daughter's wedding," Dr. Brownell says. "The wedding was only a month away, and she obviously couldn't have done it. She may actually have lost 20 pounds, but she would still feel as if she failed."

The Awful Imperative is the third category. Dieters, it seems, establish strict rules for themselves, which, because of normal human nature, they will inevitably break. "They tell themselves, 'I will *never* eat chocolate cake again,' or 'I will *never* stop for fries and a milkshake on the way home', or 'I will *never* buy a doughnut when the cart comes around at the office,' " Dr. Brownell says. "And when they fail, they can't forgive themselves."

Then there's number four, Dead End Thinking. It's based on envy. Overweight people fall into it when they focus on the unchangeable fact that some people seem to "eat like horses and still look like models." This form of thinking goes nowhere.

Why establish these four categories? To provide dieters with mental first aid, Dr. Brownell says. Whenever they feel anxious or guilty, they can stop and ask themselves whether their racing thoughts belong in one of the categories. Thoughts that do fit one of the four descriptions can be dismissed as irrational.

Try to "Think Thin"

Sometimes, however, positive thought patterns aren't enough—it takes positive imagery to reinforce them and make them more effective. Hypertensives lower their blood pressure with thoughts of Hawaii, and cancer patients envision their white cells. In a similar way, overweight people can, to some extent, get thin by thinking thin.

"We ask them to imagine themselves lighter," says psychologist Peter Miller, Ph.D., clinical psychologist and executive director of the Hilton Head Health Institute in South Carolina. He believes that building confidence and self-esteem is more important, at first, than losing pounds.

"Instead of asking them to pretend that they are already at their ideal weight, which could be discouraging, we tell them to imagine that they are about 20 pounds lighter. Then we tell them to close their eyes and see themselves standing in front of a mirror with a bathing suit on, looking the way they'd like to look," Dr. Miller says.

"Then we ask them to imagine how it would feel to be shopping for flattering clothes or to be working in an office or to be in certain family situations. It's important for them to visualize themselves behaving differently rather than just appearing different."

Images as mental tools are also important to Suki Rappaport, Ph.D., director of the Transformations Institute in Mill Valley, California. She believes that people with a positive attitude can make over their lives against great odds. To help her overweight clients, she has created two images. For lack of formal names, call one the nourishment pie and the other the human tape deck.

If you're serious about controlling your weight, she says, draw a circle and prepare to divide it up as if it were a pie. Pretend that it represents all of the various ways in which you can give yourself physical or emotional nourishment. If you are someone who can't lose weight, that pie may, at the moment, be filled with nothing but food.

Dr. Rappaport asks her clients to identify every potential source of nourishment and tells them to give each one a proportionate slice of the pie. If they like swimming, they should give swimming a slice that reflects its importance to them. If they like films, theatergoing should get a slice. Using this image, Dr. Rappaport shows people, in a very positive way, that food isn't their only source of pleasure.

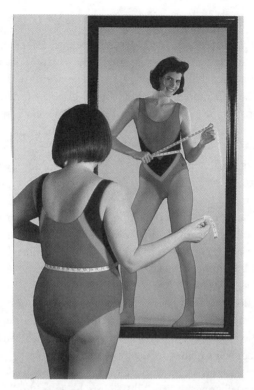

"Imagine yourself thinner" is the advice that some experts give people who want to lose weight. This kind of positive imagery is a strong motivational factor in successful weight-loss programs.

She also asks her clients to imagine that their bodies are cassette tape recorders and that each of their customary ways of responding to the world is represented by a different tape. She says that overweight people too often reach for the "binge" tape when they become anxious. Ideally, in her opinion, overweight people should get rid of their eating tape and come up with a tape that is more constructive.

"We try to say 'yes' to positive, life-affirming things, rather than 'no, no, no' to negative things," Dr. Rappaport explains. "Then people realize, 'I could have gotten a great massage with the time and money I spent eating.' This approach gives people new options."

Clothes Make the Man and Woman

Clothing, interestingly, can have symbolic value for someone who is trying to lose weight. Max Rosenbaum, Ph.D., a New York psychologist, has found that men and women who have been losing and gaining for many years often accumulate a closet full of clothes of many different sizes. A man may have shirts with necks of 15, 16 and 17 inches, and a woman might have dresses from size 7 to 13 and from "junior" to "misses."

"One woman we know spent her adolescence swinging back and forth, gaining weight and losing it," says Dr. Rosenbaum, who runs an obesity treatment program at New York's American Short-Term Therapy Center, which he and a colleague founded. "As a result, she never gained a clear image of herself. Her closet was full of clothes of different sizes, depending on her measurements at the moment, and these clothes prevented her from gaining a stable self-image. 'If I am fat today and skinny tomorrow,' she would think, 'then who am I? Which is the real me?' "

Dr. Miller's patients have run into the same sort of problem. He deals with it this way. "We tell people to throw away their bigger sizes," he says. "They've got to cut down to one size of clothes. We say, if they intend to keep their weight down, why keep those clothes? We know that as long as those clothes are in the closet, they will have doubts about their ability to change, and they'll be more likely to slip." In this way, clothes change from being a negative incentive into a positive incentive.

Yet another way to develop a positive self-image is simply to start reaching out to other people. "I tell my overweight women patients to start saying nice things to their husbands and children and start thinking positively about their friends," says Aileen B. Ludington, M.D., of Los Angeles, who once battled a weight problem of her own. "People find that if they can make other people happy, then their own self-image improves. I ask them to make a list of the things they like about their spouses and children. If you write things down, it's easier to visualize a problem. And it works for them. They come back with stories about how much their families are responding to them."

Fat Insulates the Psyche

Within the field of psychotherapy, there is an approach to solving weight problems that is significantly different from the ones mentioned so far. Many psychiatrists, for example, believe that overeating is self-destructive behavior, and they treat it as a symptom of self-hate. Overeaters use food to comfort themselves when they are unhappy, the theory goes. They do so because it is less painful to raid the refrigerator than to unearth the emotional roots of their unhappiness.

"Food is a basic form of oral gratification, an immature method of finding security. And when people are agitated, eating helps them feel better," says Dr. Rosenbaum. "People use their weight as a defense against upsetting problems. Their fat acts as insulation against hurt."

"Staying fat can become very comfortable. The idea of losing weight and actually becoming thin would present a whole new set of problems," says Mildred Klingman, a New York psychotherapist and author of the book *The Secret Lives of Fat People.*

"People who are overweight are very sensitive people," adds Dr. Rappaport. "They can sense dishonesty, and when they do, they retreat into a system that they have control over. They can control the size of their bodies. And their fat gives them a buffer zone."

Overweight young women have mothers who habitually criticize their appearance, psychiatrists say. In many cases, the same mother once urged her daughter to "eat, eat, eat" for good health. This situation made the girl angry with herself and her mother. Overeating supplies an outlet for the anger.

"One young woman we know got even with her mother by overeating," says Milton Berger, M.D., who founded the American Short-Term Therapy Center with Dr. Rosenbaum. "She knew how upset her mother would get. There's a certain satisfaction to that, a vindictive satisfaction in triumphing over others. At the same time, she is really only hurting herself."

Dr. Brownell takes issue with the emphasis of this approach. He believes that some professionals err in suggesting that the majority of overweight people have emotional problems and that they need to resolve their repressed conflicts before they can solve their eating problems.

"Some professionals tell people that they are maladjusted," he says. "So many overweight people fall prey to the idea that they hate themselves and that they are stuck in an immature stage of development. This is counterproductive."

Which technique, then, works best: learning not to fall into one of

Dr. Brownell's four negative thought patterns, or remembering not to plug a "binge" cassette into your metaphorical tape deck, or searching your childhood for the source of the problem? The answer can only be that different therapies work for different people. But it's clear that change can't take place until each overweight person upgrades his self-image.

Indeed, self-love is apparently the only way out. "Overweight people must learn to respect their bodies," Dr. Rosenbaum says. "That's very basic to successful weight loss. Overeating is closely related to poor self-concept. And when they begin to go through withdrawal, as all overweight people do, they have to say to themselves, 'I respect my body. I respect my body. I want to live.' "

Help Your Body Melt Fat

If you're overweight, you know it's no small injustice. Your reed-slim friend can win a pie-eating contest and not gain an ounce. You, on the other hand, seem to put on five pounds just thinking about pie.

You have a sneaking suspicion that your metabolism is out of whack, but you don't dare suggest it. Most medical experts regard "It's my metabolism" as a lame cover-up for all those second helpings you obviously helped yourself to and the chocolate bars they're sure you've got stashed away in your desk drawer.

But these days they're not so quick to prescribe a diet and a dose of guilt. It truly may not be your fault. Recent studies, still controversial, indicate that all metabolisms are not created equal. Your skinny pie-eating friend may have a metabolism that allows her to burn up all those excess calories as heat while yours stores them as fat.

Don't be alarmed, though. You're not doomed. There's evidence you can get your metabolism revved up by new patterns and combinations of exercise, diet and everyday habits. Why? To take advantage of a still-mysterious metabolic phenomenon called dietary-induced thermogenesis.

Though quite a mouthful, it simply means that your body generates heat after you've eaten. That's why you often push away from a large meal feeling uncomfortably warm. You can get that same feeling after exercise, and, of course, that's no coincidence. Something similar is happening.

Turning Up the Heat

When you exercise, your body is burning up calories. The digestive process is a calorie-burning activity, too. After a meal, the body works hard to store what you've eaten as fuel. Though it retains some food energy as fat, it gives off some as heat. And the more you burn off as heat, the less you store as fat.

Some of the latest research has shown that overweight people many times do not eat more than their thinner counterparts. They simply have sluggish metabolisms that don't generate that slimming after-dinner blaze. And dieting doesn't help. Their efficient, fat-storing metabolisms regard even a moderate caloric cutback as a signal that starvation is at hand, and they begin to store fat in case the food shortage goes on indefinitely.

But here's the real news. Exercise can fan the flames of even a "sluggish" metabolism—in at least four different ways. The *timing* of your meals and your exercise can also help your slimming program.

Peter M. Miller, Ph.D., director of the Hilton Head Health Institute in South Carolina, teaches his clients to pare off the pounds by fanning those fires. The double whammy of *The Hilton Head Metabolism Diet* is a combination of a low-calorie but four-meal-a-day diet and moderate but well-timed exercise.

The aim of the Hilton Head Diet is to get those fires stoked and keep them burning all day long. Dr. Miller says he divided his low-calorie diet into four meals to take advantage of the after-meal thermic effect. After all, digestion burns up calories. And before the blaze becomes a pile of embers, Dr. Miller recommends a brisk 20-minute walk. If done no later than 20 minutes after at least two meals a day, your postmeal heat production can be enhanced by up to 50 percent, he says. So, if your digestive processes normally burn 100 calories, a brisk walk for 20 minutes could increase that to 150. Do that after two meals each day and that's 36,500 calories a year—more than ten pounds of fat. "Exercise after meals burns calories more efficiently than any other exercise schedule," Dr. Miller says. "It's at this time that you're primed to increase your metabolic rate. So step on the gas. Take advantage of this maximum time."

Once you master two brisk walks a day, you might want to consider graduating to more aerobic exercises. Researchers at the University of New Hampshire found that an increase in aerobic capacity (your body's ability to use oxygen) significantly increases the number of calories you burn after a meal—even if you're *not* exercising at that particular time.

The Benefits of Aerobic Exercise

When they tested dietary-induced thermogenesis in a group of men and women, they discovered that those with greater capacity burned more calories after eating (or, in this case, drinking high- and low-calorie drinks). And the men (but not the women) were more likely to have a lower percentage of body fat. The best news, however, is that those not-terribly-fit people who improved their aerobic capacity by exercise were *also* able to stoke their after-meal blaze. One woman who increased her aerobic capacity by only 15 percent boosted her heat response by 110 percent.

Not everyone is going to be able to achieve the aerobic fitness of a well-conditioned athlete. Many athletes have metabolisms that allow them to burn hundreds of calories while doing nothing more strenuous than watching television. Aerobic capacity can be increased only within limits because it largely depends on the number of muscle fibers you're born with. But, though you can't add muscle fibers, you can make the ones you have more effective through aerobic exercise.

Jogging, tennis, dancing—anything that gets your heart pumping and your muscles moving and forces your body to break down fat for energy—can increase your aerobic capacity. Aerobic exercise for 30 minutes three times a week will stimulate your metabolism so that you'll burn calories at a faster rate than usual for as long as 24 hours after exercise—*in addition* to the hundreds you'll be burning during the exercise. "Aerobic activity stimulates the metabolism better than any other factor," says Dr. Miller.

It does something else, too. It increases your muscle mass at the same time it reduces the amount of fat you're carrying. People who have a high ratio of muscle to fat have higher metabolic rates. They can eat more and not gain weight because they burn more, even when they're sleeping.

"The reason for this is that muscle tissue is metabolically more active than fat tissue," Dr. Miller says. "It takes more body energy for muscle to function. Fat is relatively inactive, while muscle cells are

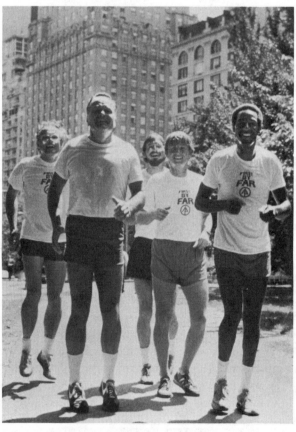

These people are obviously enjoying their jog in the park. But they are also increasing their metabolic rate. Later, when they are back at their desks, they will continue to burn more calories than if they hadn't run on their lunch hour.

extremely active, even when you are resting. A muscle furnace is constantly burning food fuel at a rapid rate day after day."

So to review, exercise can boost your metabolism in at least three different ways—in addition to the immediate calorie burnoff. First, when exercise follows a meal, it increases dietary thermogenesis—"roasting" calories that would otherwise be stored as fat. Second, regular aerobic exercise increases metabolism all day long—giving an extra boost after meals even if you're just reading a book. And third, by adding muscle, with its high metabolic rate, you're subtracting extra calories from your system every moment of the day.

How to Fan the Fires

But exercise and meal timing aren't the only factors that affect your metabolism. What you eat, even the temperature of your home, can either fan the fires or hose them down.

Make smart food choices. Eat more fruits, vegetables and whole grains, the complex carbohydrates. Avoid fats and simple carbohydrates (candy, soft drinks, desserts). Elliot Danforth Jr., M.D., director of the Clinical Research Center at the University of Vermont, says a return "to the diet of our ancestors" can have a significant impact on obesity. That means a diet that is about two-thirds complex carbohydrates and the rest protein and fat. Why? "There's a clear biochemical reason for this," says Dr. Danforth, who did many of the early studies on metabolism and obesity. "You expend only about 3 percent of your fat calories storing them as fat, but you expend 25 percent of your carbohydrate calories storing them as fat. The metabolic cost is far higher to store carbohydrates as fat. Any Iowa pig farmer will tell you. When you ask him how he gets his pigs so fat, he'll tell you it isn't by feeding them wheat, it's by feeding them fat."

Take advantage of climate control. Extremes of heat or cold increase your metabolism by as much as 10 percent, says Dr. Miller. Even a small deviation helps. Set your thermostat at 68°F in the winter and 79°F in the summer. You'll get used to the temperatures and your metabolism will get a boost.

Like most sensible weight-loss regimens, this is a lifetime proposition. Once you perk up your metabolism, it will be your ally. But you've got to keep it perked up through diet and exercise.

Get Your Mate to Help You Lose Weight

Susan looks in the mirror and groans, "I am definitely going on a diet."

"It never worked before, what makes you think it will work this time?" her husband, Bob, quickly retorts.

And then, later that same evening, he eats ice cream directly in front of her, knowing full well that ice cream is the one thing she can never resist.

The next day he suggests they go out to dinner at her favorite, fattening restaurant.

"What's the use?" she says to herself. "I might as well not even try."

Yet there is hope. Susan may be able to get Bob to stop sabotaging her diet and actually help her lose weight.

Ultimately, the success of a diet doesn't depend on your spouse, it depends on you. But in some cases, having a supportive person around makes the difference between a diet that works and one that doesn't, says Kelly Brownell, Ph.D., associate professor in the Department of Psychiatry at the University of Pennsylvania School of Medicine and co-director of the Obesity Research Clinic. Diet saboteurs may have several concerns, says Dr. Brownell, who is the author of *The LEARN Program for Weight Control.* "They may fear you will become too attractive to the opposite sex, you'll make more physical and emotional demands, you'll make new friends and have a social life that excludes them, or that you might become more competitive and independent," he says.

Getting the Right Kind of Support

Even when mates want to help, they may not know how, says Dr. Brownell. And so they take on the role of policeman, catching violations and doling out warnings. That can make matters worse. You get angry and tell your mate to mind his or her own business, or you feel like a failure and eat even more.

The other person's negative comments may be his or her way of trying to help. But no one's forcing you to eat. You always have a choice.

You may find the strength to make the right choice despite those negative comments if you think more highly of yourself and put yourself first a little more, says Peter Miller, Ph.D., clinical psychologist and executive director of the Hilton Head Health Institute in South Carolina.

"You may need to take more time for activities that make you feel good. That could mean taking time away from other things, delegating responsibilities and getting some cooperation from your family," he says. And that's not always easy.

Your mate might agree, "You need to take more time for yourself, you need to exercise." But then as soon as you start to do it, he or she will say, "Just do this one thing for me first." So you have to stand your ground and take the time for yourself, says Dr. Miller.

If your mate seems threatened every time you decide to slim down, some reassurance may ease his or her mind, says Dr. Brownell. Sue could explain to Bob that she doesn't like the feeling that food controls her, she wants her clothes to fit better and she wants to feel more energetic. All the while, she needs to continue showing she loves him and keep from implying that he is responsible for her weight problem.

There are a number of other ways you can get your mate on your side, says Dr. Brownell. "The first is to communicate. Let him know that you'd like some help." Get a reading on your spouse's feelings about your weight problem, and talk about how to best proceed.

Let your mate know what kind of help you need. Do you want to be praised when you do well or scolded when you do poorly? Should your mate avoid eating when you're around? Can he or she help by exercising with you?

Make specific suggestions about how your partner can help, leaving nothing to chance. Don't say, "Will you please help me?" Instead say, "It helps me a lot when you walk with me after dinner," or "I appreciate it when you don't eat ice cream in front of me at night."

Make the request positive. A negative request would be, "It makes it difficult for me to stick to my diet when you eat ice cream in front of

Rate Your Mate

This quiz, developed by Kelly Brownell, Ph.D., will help you evaluate whether your partner is supportive. Answer each question, add the numbers beside the responses you checked, then use the scoring guide that follows.

1. It is easy to talk to my partner about weight.
True _____ (5) False _____ (1)

2. My partner has always been thin and does not understand my weight problem. True _____ (3) False _____ (1)

3. My partner offers me food when he or she knows I am on a diet. True _____ (1) False _____ (5)

4. My partner never says critical things about my weight.
True _____ (3) False _____ (1)

5. My partner is always there when I need a friend.
True _____ (4) False _____ (1)

6. When I lose weight and look better, my partner will be jealous. True _____ (1) False _____ (3)

me." A positive request would be, "Please help me by not eating ice cream in front of me." Positive statements make people feel good, and they respond better.

Finally, make sure you reward your partner for helping you. Don't expect the support and encouragement to flow only from your mate to you. Some of it has to flow back, says Dr. Brownell. Being supportive can be draining, so you need to acknowledge your partner's help. You've been receiving help, so do some nice things in return. There are many pleasurable rewards that you can give to your partner. Send flowers, buy your mate a new record, make Sunday breakfast, fix something that's broken, see the city or give your partner a massage.

If being direct and discussing how your partner's behavior makes you feel doesn't turn your mate from a saboteur into a supporter,

7. My partner will be genuinely interested in helping me with my weight. True _____ (6) False _____ (1)

8. I could talk to my partner even if I was doing poorly. True _____ (5) False _____ (1)

Scoring

If you scored between 30 and 34, you may have found the perfect partner. A score in this range indicates that you and your mate are comfortable with one another and can work together.

If you scored between 25 and 29, your mate is potentially a good diet partner, but there are a few areas of concern. Try asking your partner to take the quiz and predict how you answered the questions. This may help you make a decision.

If you scored between 17 and 24, there are potential areas of conflict, and a diet partnership could encounter stormy going.

If you scored between 8 and 16, a diet partnership in this case would be a high-risk undertaking. Consider an alternate source of support, such as a friend, co-worker or relative.

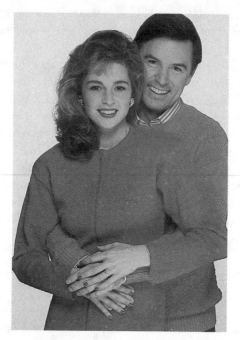

A supportive mate can make the difference between a diet that works and one that doesn't. If you want to lose those extra pounds more easily, you should discuss with your partner what he or she can do to help.

then the best thing is to ignore it and get on with your diet, says Dr. Brownell.

When the other person heads for the ice cream, you may have to walk out the door and take a walk around the block. Or call a friend on the phone and start talking to get your mind off what's making you want to eat.

Giving Support

If you are in the role of supporter, how should you behave? Be upbeat and encouraging, says Dr. Brownell. You can say, "You look good, I'm proud of you," but don't push yourself on the other person. Ask your mate what type of encouragement he or she needs and how often. You may be surprised by what kind of help the dieter wants, says Dr. Brownell.

If your mate slips up a little and happens to eat something that's forbidden or doesn't exercise, don't respond with sarcasm or negative comments such as "There you go again," or "You know you shouldn't be eating that." Learn to forgive and forget lapses.

You could be supportive by exercising with your mate. Take daily walks together or develop new interests that you can share.

Help out more. Make dinner or offer to get the kids ready for bed so your mate can go for a walk.

Be easy to please. Eat the same kind of foods so you don't have to fix two different kinds of dinners every night.

For more tips on successful dieting, alone or with a partner, you can order a copy of Dr. Brownell's book, *The LEARN Program for Weight Control,* by sending a check for $18 to Dr. Kelly Brownell, Department of Psychiatry, University of Pennsylvania, 133 South 36th Street, Philadelphia, PA 19104. Bulk rates are available.

Sip Your Way to Slimness

Which has more calories: a nut-filled brownie or an accompanying glass of milk? A mug of beer or a whiskey sour? A glass of orange juice or a glass of Coca-Cola?

If you don't have a clue, it's probably because you're not used to thinking about the calorie content of beverages. After all, solid food is where most of the world's calories lurk, right? Serious weight watchers fret about the fattening possibilities of gingerbread cakes, pumpkin pies and oversized eclairs. But who cares about liquid calories?

Maybe we all should. For some people, beverages may account for close to 50 percent of total calorie intake. For most of us, the percentage is probably far higher than we think. And there are scores of drinks with higher calorie counts than any of the sinfully caloric desserts mentioned above. Besides, it's easier to substitute a low-calorie beverage for a high-calorie one if you know where all the calories are. (See the table, Beverage Caloric Guide, on page 50.)

How to Cut
Your Alcohol Calories

Although alcoholic beverages, especially beer and some mixed drinks, are notoriously high in calories, it *is* possible to lose weight without forsaking alcohol completely. Here's how.

At cocktail parties and bars.   Whether you're just "having a few" with some friends or celebrating a special occasion, the following tips will help you control how much you drink.

- Stop early. Cocktail *hour* is a misnomer—most of them last a lot longer. Set a cutoff time for yourself, or stop when you start to feel the liquor. Drink only nonalcoholic beverages after that. Better yet, schedule something for afterward that forces you to leave early.
- Switch back and forth. An alternative to stopping: Follow every drink with a glass of water. You'll always have something in your hand to sip, but you'll be getting half the liquor and calories. You'll also counteract alcohol's dehydrating actions. And a dry body is what causes the dreaded hangover.
- Dilute your drink. Start out with a regular drink, but when it's half gone, add water or club soda to it. Every time your glass is half empty again, add more water or soda.
- Duck the waiter. Never order a drink from that roving drink machine. Go to the bar and order it yourself. Chances are you'll be so involved in conversation, your trips will be limited.
- Sip slowly. A warm martini, a flat gin and tonic or a diluted Bloody Mary isn't very appealing. The longer your drink lasts, the less you'll feel like finishing it.
- Fix a drink you don't like. Some punches are so delicious that you can gulp down several glasses without thinking about it. If this happens to you, try ordering a bitter drink that doesn't appeal to you. You'll probably drink less of it.

In restaurants.   When dining out, it's sometimes easy to drink more than you realize: a cocktail before dinner, wine with the meal, maybe brandy afterward. Here are some suggestions for cutting down.

- Arrive early. Let's say you don't want to drink alcohol but you don't want your friends to rib you about it. You can head these people off at the pass by arriving early and ordering a well-disguised nonalcoholc drink. If your friend wants to order a second round, you can simply tell the waiter you'll have another of "the same."
- Order food first, drinks second. This way, you'll probably have time for only one drink before the meal is served.
- Dine with fine wine. Order only one bottle of very fine wine and savor it slowly before and during your meal. You probably won't want to pay the extra cost of ordering more, and you will enjoy it more.

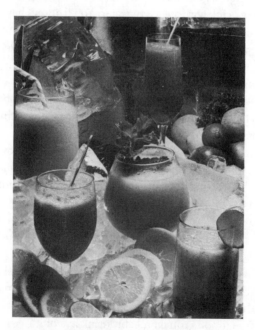

It's easy to overlook the calories in beverages. If you're trying to lose weight, however, you should be especially aware of what they add to your daily total.

Learning Where the Calories Hide

Are you curious about the answers to the mini-quiz at the beginning of the chapter? Well, a glass of whole milk packs 159 calories, while a brownie has only 97; a mug of regular beer has about 150 calories, a whiskey sour 184; and a glass of orange juice carries 84 calories, while a glass of Coca-Cola has 72.

If those figures are different from what you expected, take a look at the table on the following pages for more surprises. Our information comes from government nutrition data banks, manufacturers and, in some cases, from laboratory analyses carried out for this report.

Here's to a wiser and slimmer you!

Beverage Caloric Guide

Beverage	Serving Size (fl. oz.)	Calories per Serving (approx.)	Calories per Ounce (approx.)
Fruit Juices			
Apple cider	8	118	15
Apple juice	8	118	15
Knudsen cherry cider	8	96	12
Apricot nectar	7	125	18
Guava nectar	6	300	50
Pear nectar	5½	100	18
Knudsen papaya nectar	8	104	13
Libby's peach nectar	6	90	15
Cranapple juice, low-calorie	8	43	5
Cranapple juice, regular	8	173	22
Cranberry juice cocktail, low-calorie	8	48	6
Cranberry juice cocktail, regular	8	141	18
Crangrape juice	8	144	18
Cranprune juice	8	154	19

(continued)

Beverage Caloric Guide—*Continued*

Beverage	Serving Size (fl. oz.)	Calories per Serving (approx.)	Calories per Ounce (approx.)
Fruit Juices—*continued*			
Grape juice	8	170	21
Prune juice	4	92	23
Grapefruit juice, canned	8	101	13
Grapefruit juice, fresh	8	96	12
Knudsen pink grapefruit juice	8	76	10
Limeade, from frozen concentrate	8	100	13
Lime juice, from concentrate	1	4	4
Lemon juice	1	6	6
Orange juice, canned, unsweetened	8	120	15
Orange juice, fresh	8	112	14
Orange juice, frozen reconstituted	8	122	15
Orange juice, imitation (Awake, Bright and Early, etc.)	8	120	15
Tangerine juice	8	122	15
Five Alive juice	8	114	14
Pineapple juice, canned, unsweetened	8	138	17
Acerola juice	8	56	7
Coconut milk (liquid from mixture of coconut meat and coconut water)	8	605	76
Coconut water (liquid from coconuts)	8	53	7
Blackberry juice, canned, unsweetened	8	91	11
Tangelo juice	8	101	13
Winter Hill apple-apricot juice	6	95	16
Winter Hill apple-raspberry juice	6	88	15

Beverage	Serving Size (fl. oz.)	Calories per Serving (approx.)	Calories per Ounce (approx.)
Winter Hill apple-strawberry juice	6	88	15
Mott's apple-grape juice	8	113	14
Pineapple-orange juice	8	126	16
Pear-apple cider	8	100	13
Pear-grape juice	8	110	14
Fruit Drinks			
Orange-apricot juice drink, canned, 40% fruit juices	8	125	16
Del Monte pineapple-grapefruit juice drink	8	120	15
Del Monte pineapple-orange juice drink	8	120	15
Knudsen Hibiscus Cooler	8	94	12
Gatorade bottled drinks, all flavors	8	56	7
Hawaiian Punch canned drinks, all flavors	8	120	15
Knudsen sparkling fruit juice, strawberry	8	75	9
Hi-C canned drinks, all flavors	8	120	15
Harvest of Nature fruit punch, sugar-free	8	8	1
Ocean Spray Cran-Tastic blended juice drink	6	110	18
Country Time drink mixes, all flavors	8	88	11
Crystal Light drink mix, sugar-free, orange	8	4	0.5
Hawaiian Punch drink mix	8	104	13
Hi-C drink mixes, all flavors	8	104	13

(continued)

Beverage Caloric Guide—*Continued*

Beverage	Serving Size (fl. oz.)	Calories per Serving (approx.)	Calories per Ounce (approx.)
Fruit Drinks—*continued*			
Kool-Aid drink mixes, all flavors except lemonade	8	104	13
Kool-Aid drink mixes, sugar-free, all flavors	8	4	0.5
Tang drink mixes, all flavors	8	120	15
Gatorade drink mixes, all flavors	8	56	7
Kool-Aid lemonade drink mix	8	104	13
Crystal Light lemonade mix	8	4	0.5
Wyler's lemonade drink mix	8	88	11
Lemonade, from frozen concentrate	8	107	14
Coffee and Tea			
Tea, clear	8	2	0.3
Tea, instant, sweetened	8	86	11
Tea, instant, unsweetened	8	0	0
Celestial Seasonings Red Zinger herb tea	6	1	0.2
Coffee, black	8	2.7	0.3
Coffee, instant, black	8	1.3	0.2
General Foods International Coffee, Irish Mocha Mint	8	67	8
Magic Mountain instant herb tea	8	4	0.5
Postum cereal beverage	6	12	2
Vegetable Drinks			
Tomato juice	8	46	6
Tomato juice cocktail	8	51	6
V-8 vegetable juice cocktail	8	52	7
Carrot juice	8	93	12

Beverage	Serving Size (fl. oz.)	Calories per Serving (approx.)	Calories per Ounce (approx.)
Mott's Beefamato	8	97	12
Mott's Clamato	8	114	14
Knudsen Very Veggie	8	32	4
Beer			
Augsberger	12	175	15
Beck's dark	12	156	13
Beck's light	12	132	11
Birell Premium Light nonalcohol malt beverage	12	75	6
Budweiser	12	150	13
Busch	12	156	13
Coors	12	142	12
Coors Light	12	102	9
Dos Equis amber	12	144	12
Foster's lager	12	120	10
Gablinger's	12	96	8
Guinness Extra Stout	12	192	16
Hamm's	12	136	11
Heineken	12	152	13
Heineken Special Dark	12	192	16
Hofbrau dark reserve	12	204	17
Hofbrau light reserve	12	144	12
Kirin	12	149	12
Kronenbourg	12	170	14
Lowenbrau	12	157	13
Michelob	12	163	14
Michelob Light	12	134	11
Miller High Life	12	150	13
Miller Lite	12	96	8
Natural Light	12	110	9
Newcastle Brown Ale	12	144	12

(continued)

Beverage Caloric Guide—*Continued*

Beverage	Serving Size (fl. oz.)	Calories per Serving (approx.)	Calories per Ounce (approx.)
Beer—*continued*			
Pabst Blue Ribbon	12	150	13
Schlitz	12	148	12
Schlitz Light	12	96	8
St. Pauli Girl light	12	144	12
St. Pauli Girl dark	12	156	13
Stroh Boch	12	157	13
Stroh Bohemian	12	148	12
Stroh Light	12	115	10
Texas Select nonalcohol malt beverage	12	65	5
Wurzburger Hofbrau nonalcohol malt beverage	12	111	9
Wine			
California brand wine cooler	3½	20	6
Carl Jung dealcoholed white wine	3	20	7
Champagne	3½	71	20
Dessert, sweet	3½	153	44
Fu-Ki saki	1½	36	24
Harvey's Bristol Cream	3½	207	59
Martinelli's sparkling cider	6	100	17
Masson light rose	3½	54	15
Port	3	134	45
Red table	3½	76	22
Sherry	3½	147	42
Taylor California Cellars Light	3½	55	16
Vermouth, dry	3½	105	30
Vermouth, sweet	3½	184	53
White table	3½	80	23

Beverage	Serving Size (fl. oz.)	Calories per Serving (approx.)	Calories per Ounce (approx.)
Hard Drinks			
Bailey's Original Irish Cream	1	85	85
Brandy	1	69	69
Cordials, liqueur	1	97	97
Daiquiri	3½	122	35
Gin, rum, vodka, whiskey (80 proof)	1½	97	65
Gin, rum, vodka, whiskey (86 proof)	1½	105	70
Gin, rum, vodka, whiskey (90 proof)	1½	110	74
Gin, rum, vodka, whiskey (94 proof)	1½	116	77
Gin, rum, vodka, whiskey (100 proof)	1½	124	83
Jose Cortez tequila (80 proof)	1½	36	24
Kahlúa	1	119	119
Manhattan	3¼	233	72
Martini	2½	152	61
Whiskey sour	3½	184	53
Soft Drinks			
Quinine soda	12	113	9
Club soda	12	0	0
Dad's root beer	12	158	13
Shasta root beer	12	164	14
Hires root beer	12	150	13
Old Tyme ginger beer	12	160	13
Faygo old-fashioned root beer, sugar-free	8	0	0
Dr. Brown's orange soda	12	174	15

(continued)

Beverage Caloric Guide—*Continued*

Beverage	Serving Size (fl. oz.)	Calories per Serving (approx.)	Calories per Ounce (approx.)
Soft Drinks—*continued*			
Shasta orange soda	12	128	11
Dr. Brown's cream soda	12	162	14
A-Treat cream soda	12	126	11
Old Tyme cream soda	12	160	13
Old Tyme apple soda	12	160	13
Moxie soda	12	180	15
Yoo Hoo chocolate drink	12	180	15
Bitter Lemon	6	96	16
Pepsi	12	158	13
Diet Pepsi	12	0	0
Coca-Cola	12	144	12
Diet Coke	12	0	0
A-Treat cola, sugar-free	12	6	0.5
Dr. Pepper	12	144	12
7-Up	12	146	12
Diet 7-Up	12	4	0.3
Mountain Dew	12	178	15
Milk Drinks			
Whole milk, 3.5% fat	8	159	20
Low-fat milk, 2% fat	8	120	15
Low-fat milk, 1% fat	8	102	13
Low-fat milk, 1% fat, lactose reduced	8	100	13
Skim milk	8	86	11
Buttermilk	8	99	12
Goat's milk	8	168	21
Eggnog (no alcohol)	4	171	43
Malted milk, chocolate	8	233	29
Chocolate milk, whole	8	208	26
Hot cocoa	8	218	27
Carnation hot cocoa mix, regular	6	110	18

Beverage	Serving Size (fl. oz.)	Calories per Serving (approx.)	Calories per Ounce (approx.)
Carnation hot cocoa mix, sugar-free	6	50	8
Swiss Miss chocolate mix, sugar-free	8	130	16
Nestlé Quik chocolate milk mix	8	245	31
Nestlé Quik chocolate milk mix, sugar-free	8	140	18
Burger King vanilla shake	16	340	21
Burger King chocolate shake	16	340	21
McDonald's vanilla shake	16	352	22
McDonald's chocolate shake	16	383	24
Hardee's milkshake	16	391	24
Dairy Queen chocolate shake, regular	16	710	44
Ovaltine, whole milk	8	221	28
Kefir, from whole milk	8	168	21

Miscellaneous

Beverage	Serving Size (fl. oz.)	Calories per Serving (approx.)	Calories per Ounce (approx.)
Ah Soy nondairy beverage, chocolate	6	149	25
Soy Moo nondairy beverage, plain	6	98	16
Ah Soy nondairy beverage, vanilla	6	142	24
Clam juice	8	20	3
Herb Ox instant beef broth	6	6	1
Herb Ox instant chicken broth	6	6	1
Mineral water	8	0	0
Pero instant cereal beverage	6	3.2	0.5
Tonic water	12	132	11
Coco Goya piña colada mixer*	3	456	154

*1 piña colada = 3 mugs of Budweiser. Serving for serving, piña coladas are the most caloric alcoholic drinks in the world, tipping the scales at up to 450 calories or more each.

Eat Out and Lose Weight

What dieter doesn't suffer from "restaurant anxiety"—the crippling fear of blowing weeks of weight control in one madcap indulgence? Well, fear no more. With a little menu savvy, you can dodge and weave your way through just about any eatery and emerge with your waistline intact.

We know. We've reviewed scores of menus from a wide array of restaurants, comparing calorie data. What we discovered may surprise you: lots of delightfully satisfying low-calorie choices (even at eateries that traditionally serve fattening fare). Our recommendations, which follow, are based on U.S. Department of Agriculture calorie counts for standard servings. (Keep in mind that portions and recipes do vary widely from one eating establishment to another.)

Here then, the good, the bad and the best dinner choices for the calorie conscious.

Seafood Restaurant

The restaurant of choice for many dieters, seafood houses sometimes serve up deceptively fattening fare. A dozen steamed clams doesn't sound like much. But dunked in butter, they can add up to nearly 300 calories. And that's just the appetizer.

Similarly, a "low-calorie" entrée like flounder stuffed with crabmeat can easily top 500 calories if it's smothered with white sauce. Beware, too, of seafood dishes with fancy last names, such as Lobster Newburg (725 calories) or Clams Casino (550). And steer clear of combination platters. These king-size dinners often feature fried fish and high-calorie concoctions such as deviled crab or crab cakes.

Better alternatives: Take tomato-based Manhattan clam chowder over the creamy New England version and save half the calories (about 80 per cup). For similar savings, choose a clear seafood gumbo over a smooth and creamy seafood bisque. Shrimp cocktail (at 100 calories for five large shrimp with cocktail sauce) is the obvious choice over steamed clams with butter. An eight-ounce lobster tail, at just 115 calories, or six steamed whole hardshell crabs, at 144, are fine dinner entrées if you can do without the butter. If you can't, stick to broiled white fish, such as flounder, scrod or haddock, moistened with lemon juice.

Best bet: "Pick and peel" shrimp with cocktail sauce. Beyond the obvious caloric advantage, any seafood—such as shrimp in the shell, stone-crab claws or steamed hardshell crabs—that you must first pry from its shell slows eating to an appetite-satisfying pace.

Our entrée recommendation is grilled kabob of shrimp, scallops or white fish and vegetables at 230 calories per serving.

American Steak House

A juicy steak, the dieter's choice of years gone by, has fallen from favor. The reason: Many cuts of beef are high in fat, and fat is high in calories. Generally, the better the cut, the more calories from fat. Filet mignon, Delmonico and New York strip steaks owe their tenderness to fat marbling. Beware, too, of steak-house toppings such as mushrooms, onions or peppers. They are usually sautéed in butter.

Better alternatives: From a calorie standpoint, London broil is a cut above the rest. At 477 calories for a generous (but often standard) eight-ounce portion, it contains up to 200 calories less per serving than the steaks mentioned. Another calorie-miser tip: Order your meat cooked to medium-well; the longer the meat cooks, the more fat is rendered from it.

Best bet: Cut your steak in half; offer the other half to your tableside partner or take it home for another meal. Then center your meal around other standard steak-house items: salad and baked potato. Ask for some low-calorie salad dressing on the side to sprinkle over your greens and potato (instead of sour cream or butter).

American Diner

On the downside, diners tend to serve many precooked dishes, such as meat loaf and chicken croquettes, that are loaded with fattening fillers. Made-to-order items are often grilled in grease or fried.

Better alternatives: Roast turkey, at 132 calories without gravy, or broiled haddock or flounder, at 117 without butter, are standard on every diner menu. Ordering mashed potatoes (without gravy or butter) instead of bread stuffing saves you another 200 calories. For an appetizer, choose a half grapefruit or a melon wedge (each less than 50 calories) over fruit cup, which may carry the extra weight of a sugary syrup. Or have a glass of tomato juice. At 21 calories, it has about half the caloric clout of orange or apple juice and less than a quarter of grape juice.

Best bet: Create a 1980s' grazing experience in a 1950s' diner setting. Order a tossed salad, dressing on the side, and an assortment of vegetables. Pickled cabbage, unsweetened applesauce, string beans, corn and low-fat cottage cheese don't add up to a hill of beans, calorically speaking. But keep in mind that pickled red beets, at 90 calories a half-cup serving, are an unexpected heavy hitter.

Pizza Shop

Pizza alone is not bad: about 120 calories for a slice of thin-crust pie. It's the toppings that can spell trouble. Just four slices of pepperoni double the calories in a slice of pizza. Black olives and anchovies packed in oil also carry a hefty share of calories from fat.

Better alternatives: Top your pizza with fresh vegetables, such as onions, garlic, green and red peppers and mushrooms. Go easy on the cheese and olive oil.

Best bet: One slice of thick-crust pizza, topped with all the veggies you can eat. At about 165 satisfying calories, it has half the cheese and about 100 calories less than two slices of vegetable-topped thin-crust pizza.

Delicatessen

Think "deli" and you probably conjure up an image of dining on the biggest hot pastrami sandwich you can possibly fit between your jaws. In reality, that can cost you upward of 700 calories for six ounces of meat between two slices of rye. And you haven't tackled the "help yourself" table full of pickles, potato salad and coleslaw! Here, lunch can easily cost you your full day's allowance of calories, especially if you splurge on cheesecake for dessert.

Better alternatives: Take a friend and share a sandwich. Then "weigh" each sandwich ingredient alone and, more important, consider what they add up to. At 106 calories, three ounces of turkey meat, for example, is the clear choice over roast beef at 150. But when the roast beef is accompanied by mustard or horseradish (each about four or five calories a tablespoon) and the drier turkey meat requires mayo or Russian dressing (100 and 75 calories, respectively), the scales tip in favor of the roast beef. Final score: half of a turkey sandwich, 267 calories; roast beef, 216. For extras, opt for pickled cabbage or a great big deli pickle, which won't cost you more than ten calories. If you must indulge in dessert, choose a cheese blintz. Made with cottage cheese, it contains half as many calories as New York-style cheesecake (about 140).

Best bet: Half a deli sandwich consisting of three ounces of roast turkey, lettuce, tomato and mustard on one slice of rye (just 178 calories) or lox with tomato and onion on half a bagel (142).

Mexican Restaurant

South-of-the-border cuisine offers excellent diet fare, especially dishes that are light on meat and heavy on toppings like chopped tomato and pepper, shredded lettuce and salsa. There are two danger zones, however: fried foods and *grande* platter portions. An order of nachos (deep-fried tortilla chips topped with melted cheese and re-fried beans, often prepared with lard) will cost you about 800 calories. And there's more trouble in the main event: Entrées heaped high with guacamole, refried beans, cheese and sour cream contain *mucho* calories.

Better alternatives: Order a la carte. Pass up the crisp corn tortillas (which are fried) and request soft flour tortillas (which are baked). Hold the cheese, sour cream and guacamole for an additional calorie saving. And, instead of the lard-laden refried beans, take a side order of Mexican rice, worth about 50 calories less. Another smart choice: A bowl of chili with beans saves about 60 calories over the all-meat chili—hold the cheese, of course.

Best bet: A soft flour taco with chicken and rice, at just 300 calories, or a light burrito (soft flour tortilla filled with lettuce, tomato, chicken and salsa), about 340.

Italian Restaurant

From simple spaghetti houses to fine Northern Italian restaurants, one caution applies: Watch out for olive oil. A tasty but fattening ingredient (at 120 calories per tablespoon), it lurks in the garlic bread, antipasto, pesto sauce, Caesar salad, roasted sweet peppers with anchovies or tuna, and much more. Another note on fine dining: If you're intent on doing as the Romans do, be prepared for the challenge of a five-course extravaganza.

Better alternatives: For starters, choose a cup of minestrone (about 120 calories) or chicken broth with pasta (150) or an order of mussels with marinara sauce (120). Marinara, which is a meatless tomato sauce, and tomato-based red clam sauce are the lightest accompaniments to pasta. Served over a cup of spaghetti, they run about 250 calories. In the meat department, save calories by ordering chicken cacciatore, cooked in a tomato sauce, instead of chicken Parmesan, with breading and cheese. The veal dish of choice is picata, lightly sautéed with lemon. Finally, don't allow the waiter to sweet-talk you into cannoli, tortoni or spumoni. Calorie-wise, these desserts vie with the best cakes and pies America has to offer. Even the Italian ice will cost you plenty: about 250 calories.

Best bet: For a five-course meal that comes in at around 500 calories, start with melon. Next, a cup of minestrone soup, then a green salad dressed with red-wine vinegar and a fresh grinding of black pepper. Order an appetizer or child's portion of pasta with marinara sauce as an entrée. Top the meal with fresh berries and a cup of espresso.

Chinese Restaurant

The Chinese restaurant has enjoyed a reputation for light food. And therein lies the danger. Calorie-conscious diners assume everything on the menu is safe for consumption. In fact, fried rice, fried noodles, fried wontons and deep-fried egg rolls are heavyweights. Guess why.

Better alternatives: Choose chop suey over chow mein (which is traditionally served with fried noodles) for a 100-calorie-plus saving. Similarly, steamed rice is at least 50 calories less than fried rice. Hold the cornstarch for additional savings.

Best bet: Share an order of stir-fried chicken or shrimp with vegetables, served over steamed rice.

French Restaurant

First the good news: Since the French pride themselves on freshly prepared food, it's very easy for the chef to customize a dish to your diet. Now the bad news: Coaxing low-calorie fare out of a classic French chef can be an exasperating task. Fortunately, heavy cream and butter sauces are giving way to the lighter nouvelle cuisine. If your chef seems stuck in the old ways, appeal to his sense of romance: Explain that your love life is inextricably linked to your waistline.

Better alternatives: Take *salade verte* (mixed greens) over *salade Nicoise* (greens mixed with olives, eggs, tuna and anchovies) and save calories. Poached fish or quenelles (a poached fish dumpling of sorts made of pike and egg whites), or pot-au-feu (stewed chicken in broth) are excellent alternatives to the heavy, sauce-laden entrées. Know too that not all sauces are created equal: *coulis,* made of pureed vegetables, and *sauce piquante,* with tomatoes, vinegar and shallots, are calorie-miles apart from bearnaise (with egg yolks and butter), *veloute* (butter, flour and stock), bechamel (flour, butter and milk) and the crème de la crème, Mornay, made with bechamel sauce, heavy cream, egg yolks and cheese.

Best bet: Bouillabaisse—*sans aioli* (without garlic mayonnaise). This tomato- and saffron-flavored fish stew will keep you busy all night, prying mussels from their shells and lapping up every delicious drop of stock with French bread. A fabulous indulgence at just 450 calories, including the bread.

The Best Ways to Flatten Your Belly

There's nothing more disheartening. You've sweated and sacrificed to take off those 20 pounds and now, after all that work, you ought to be svelte. But, apparently, nobody has told your tummy. Your belt still looks like the equator, and you're afraid your co-workers are going to give you a surprise baby shower.

The fact is, the sensible diet and the good cardiovascular workouts that helped you melt all that fat probably did little to tone your abdominal muscles, which are the natural girdle that keeps you firm in front. They often need individual attention—exercises that build up their strength. And they need that strength for more than your good looks. The four sets of muscles that make up the abdomen, working in concert with your back muscles, help you do everything from stand upright to sit tall. Anyone who has ever had a lower-back problem knows that the first order of business to getting the back in shape is to get the abs in shape.

But you also have to get your abs in shape without wreaking havoc on your back. Some abdominal strengthening exercises are anathema to those whose back muscles are also weak. While a fit individual can do straight-leg sit-ups until the cows come home, someone not so fit may find that pain equals no gain. You want to flatten your stomach, not wind up flat on your back.

For the best and worst of the common stomach flatteners, we went to the experts. In this case we asked the advice of Charles E. Kuntzleman, Ed.D., noted fitness author; Michael Yessis, Ph.D., an Olympic trainer who teaches biomechanics and the training of athletes at California State University, Fullerton; and Steve Smith, manager of corporate health and fitness at Coca-Cola Foods in Houston, Texas. Here's what they considered the best — and worst.

(And please note, beg our experts: These exercises will not help a protruding abdomen that's the result of one too many pan pizzas. Toning exercises don't whittle away fat — only diet and aerobic exercise do that. These exercises will, however, strengthen and tighten sagging muscles, which should make you *look* as slim as you can be.)

What to Do

The Abdominal Curl.   Lying flat on the floor, keep your knees bent and your arms across your chest. Rise slowly, curling up each vertebra separately until you're at a 45-degree angle. This means your lower back should still be on the floor. Lower yourself slowly, which is a complementary exercise called the Curl-Down.

The benefits: According to Dr. Kuntzleman, who calls this "the best exercise you can do," this simple movement uses only the abdominal muscles. Because you keep your lower back firmly on the floor at all times, you don't involve weak back muscles that could be injured. (Be careful, however, not to do this with your arms behind your neck. The temptation is to pull on your neck, which could damage those muscles, warns Dr. Kuntzleman.)

The Reverse Sit-Up.   Lie flat on your back with your arms at your sides, palms down. Keep your knees bent and raise your legs and pelvis completely off the floor. In the final position, your knees will be almost above your face.

The benefits: This exercise complements the Abdominal Curl because it exercises the lower abdominals, says Dr. Yessis.

The Full Curl.   Lie flat on your back with your feet close to your buttocks, your hands behind your head. Raise your head and shoulders and lift your knees at the same time, as if your head and knees were going to meet in the middle.

The benefits: Again, you are keeping your lower back on the ground, notes Smith, who teaches this exercise to his corporate clients.

The Pelvic Tilt.   Lie flat on your back, or sit straight in a chair. Tilt your pelvis backward until your back presses against the floor or the back of the chair. Hold this position for 10 to 15 seconds, then release. Perform this exercise two or three times.

The benefits: It's an easy, simple exercise that anyone can do anywhere, says Smith.

The Reverse Trunk Twist.   Lie flat on your back, with your knees bent. Lift your legs together at a 90-degree angle, keeping your arms out to your sides. Drop your legs first to one side, then to the other.

The benefits: You're exercising your internal and external obliques, V-shaped muscle groups in the front of your abdomen that are involved in spinal flexion and rotation, says Dr. Yessis.

Isometric Toner.   You may do this standing, sitting or lying down. Simply pull your abdominal muscles inward and back toward your spine. Hold for a few seconds.

The benefits: You can do this anywhere, says Dr. Kuntzleman, and it's always safe and effective.

What Not to Do

The Straight-Leg Sit-Up.   You probably did this one in gym class. You would lie on your back, with your feet flat and your hands behind your head, then raise yourself to a sitting position. Our experts also include Bent-Knee Full Sit-Ups in the no-no category.

The disadvantages: Unless you're in good shape, chances are you'll arch your back to get all the way up. That can hurt your lower back, says Dr. Kuntzleman. Besides that, he notes, you're using your stomach muscles only half of the way up, which is why the abdominal curl is the better exercise.

The Slant-Board Sit-Up.   If you use your local gym, you know all about the slant board. To do this full sit-up, you place your feet under the padded footholds and raise yourself so you are doing a full sit-up in an inclined position.

The disadvantages: the same as Straight-Leg and Bent-Knee Sit-Ups. "I never recommend using this exercise," says Smith. "If it's done too aggressively, the hip flexor muscles are overemphasized. That can lead to pain problems."

Double Straight-Leg Raise.   This one should also be familiar. Lying flat on your back, you lift both legs off the floor to various angles and hold.

The disadvantages: Besides putting pressure on your back, says Smith, most of the work is being done by your hip flexors, not your abdominals.

How to Improve the Rotation Diet

For those of you interested in losing 1 pound or 20, consider these words from a man who has a weight-loss plan to offer: "The first thing I want to say is, don't worry! You will be able to eat again like a normal human being and not gain weight! You will be able to return to the style of cooking you prefer (unless it's loaded with fat), you will be able to eat out, and while eating out, be able to eat as others eat."

So says the originator of the best-selling Rotation Diet, and they are delicious words to both the person considering his or her first diet and to the seasoned veteran of the dieting game who's tried them all to no avail. But in a nation where diets are consumed like salted peanuts, what separates this one from the rest that have come and gone as fast as a pizza delivery boy? More important, is it a safe, nutritionally sound regimen that works?

Experts say it's not an unhealthy diet, and you will lose weight, but only in the short term. The odds are that five years after starting the diet you'll have regained the weight you lost, possibly even a few pounds more than you had when you started, and you'll join the other 80 to 95 percent of the populace who fall off the diet wagon each year.

"This isn't an outrageously bad diet like some on the market, and there are no imbalances in the vitamins and other nutrients," says psychologist Morton Harmatz, Ph.D., of the University of Massachusetts in Amherst, who's spent 15 years studying weight-loss diets and eating disorders. "It's a lot like other diets that have come and gone, though, and all of them fail in several respects: They involve strict menus that no one can adhere to for long periods of time, which is what it takes to maintain weight loss. And diets like this don't address a person's desire for food or the root causes of overeating."

The Plan

The Rotation Diet is the creation of Martin Katahn, Ph.D., a Vanderbilt University psychologist who, after losing 75 pounds 22 years ago and keeping them off, decided his weight-loss plan might just be what a diet-hungry nation needed. (It's estimated that the average American attempts 2.2 diets a year, and on any given day more than 20 million people—mostly women—are trying to lose weight.)

For the first three days of the diet, you consume only 600 calories daily. Then the calorie count jumps to 900 for each of four days. In week two, you rotate to 1,200 calories daily for seven days. (For male dieters, add 300 to the last two figures.) The third week, you're back to 600 calories (1,200 for men) each of three days, followed by four days at 900 calories each (1,500 for men). If the 600- or 900-calorie rotations leave you famished, Dr. Katahn says, jump immediately to 900 or 1,200 calories.

After this 21-day cycle, you're allowed to stop and take what Dr. Katahn labels a vacation, which is partly designed to enhance your motivation. Chances are, he says, you'll prefer not to halt the diet. His reasoning is that you'll be so pleased with the rapid weight loss, you'll want to continue slimming down. Still, he stresses that the time-out is crucial to success and insists on a week to a month off.

The vacation has limits: Don't exceed 1,200 calories a day for the first three days, or preferably a week, then move up to 1,500 calories each of three days, and then 1,800 calories daily for the remainder of your dieting hiatus. You can substitute any foods you want during this break—yes, even candy or ice cream—as long as you stay within the caloric bounds. You must drink eight eight-ounce glasses of water daily, which is also urged during the active dieting weeks. No low-calorie sodas, please, because he says they keep your taste for sweets alive.

Brisk exercise is mandatory. In Dr. Katahn's words, "If you don't get active and stay active, you've got a snowball's chance in hell of maintaining any weight loss." Dieters are to start gradually, about 15 minutes a day the first week, with brisk, vigorous exercise such as walking, swimming, gentle jogging, bicycling or bouncing on a trampo-

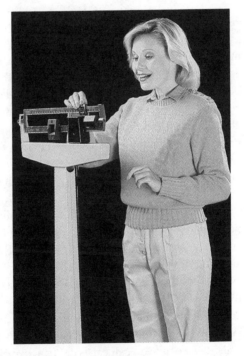

The number of calories you eat is only one of the factors to consider when you're aiming for lower numbers on the scale. Exercise, eating behavior, life-style and attitude play a large part in how successful you'll be at losing weight and keeping it off.

line. You should be up to at least 45 minutes a day by the end of the third week.

It's a mixed diet with a variety of foods, unlike the high-protein or low-carbohydrate diets that Dr. Katahn pans. Still, he advises that you may need vitamin and mineral supplements, and he stresses that anyone considering a fast weight-loss program should first consult a physician. The diet's not suitable for children and adolescents, pregnant women, nursing mothers and extremely active people, such as runners who jog miles a day.

Dr. Katahn says his diet increases your metabolic rate, which is the speed at which your body burns calories, and makes it easier to lose weight.

With most diets, the reduction in calories causes the metabolic rate to decrease. It then takes less food to create fat, and it's harder to lose the regained weight because your metabolic rate is slower than when you started dieting. (One reason for the vacation is that the slight increase in calories allowed during the break supposedly fuels the calorie-burning metabolic rate and therefore prevents it from slowing.)

Dr. Katahn allows little or no fat, sugar or salt, which may lend credence to some of the health benefit claims. He says to expect an average 10 percent reduction in serum cholesterol levels and a 15 percent drop in circulating triglycerides. People with high blood sugar are told they may see those levels normalize, and mild hypertensives might be able to reduce or eliminate blood pressure medication. The fiber in the diet's complex carbohydrates should "tangle up about 10 percent of the dietary fat you eat" so it will "pass right through your system without being digested."

You'll never get hungry on the Rotation Diet, says its originator, since you can stuff yourself with what he calls "free" vegetables — asparagus, celery, chicory, lettuce, parsley and watercress, to name a few of the 13 choices — that are low in calories but fiber and nutrient dense. There's also a list of all-you-can-eat "safe" fruits: apples, berries, grapefruit, melon, oranges, peaches, pineapple and tangerines. Pick only one type of fruit and stay with it, however, since eating several different kinds can stimulate your appetite, he warns.

On the average, expect to lose 5 pounds the first week, 2½ pounds the second week, and around 5 more pounds the third week, he says.

The heavier you are, the more you lose, and if you're more than a few pounds overweight, Dr. Katahn suggests it's not unrealistic to drop 1 pound a day during the 21-day cycle.

Computer Takes a Byte

All of which all sounds fine and good, but Kathy Musgrave was less than overwhelmed when she used a computer to compare 21 days of Rotation Diet menus with the Recommended Dietary Allowances (RDAs) for vitamins and minerals. "The diet is more than adequate for getting protein, but it's low in iron, zinc and vitamin D," says the registered dietitian, who is nutrition professor with the University of Maine-Orono School of Human Development.

The Rotation Diet supplies only 63 percent of the RDA for iron, 53 percent of the RDA for zinc and 31 percent of the RDA for vitamin D. "All the other nutrients are relatively all right," she says, "although they aren't up to 100 percent of the RDA. For example, the diet supplies 89.5 percent of the RDA for calcium for a 21-day cycle. Anything above 67 percent of the RDA is considered nutritionally safe. In any case, Dr. Katahn covers his bases by suggesting that dieters take supplements.

"Twenty-two percent of the calories in his diet come from fat, and the current national recommendation is that we get no more than 30 percent of our calories from fat, so that's a good point," she adds. "I'm concerned about the 600- and 900-calorie days, however. Even though it's only for a short while, it could be draining protein from the body's stores, so if your system is stressed or exposed to a virus, you may be more susceptible to illness.

"I'd recommend no less than 1,000 calories a day and more exercise. Instead of starting with 600 calories a day and 15 minutes of exercise, begin the diet with at least 1,000 calories daily and maybe 30 minutes of activity."

The Rotation Diet's emphasis on exercise is highly commendable, says Jennifer Anderson, a registered dietitian in the Food Science and Human Nutrition Department at Colorado State University, Fort Collins. But after studying this and other popular diets, she concludes that too little attention is paid to target heart rates.

"This is important for people in the over-50 age group, which is where a lot of dieters are, because they need special exercise programs," she says. "You don't have to get the heart beating to capacity to burn calories. You just have to speed up your metabolic rate by reaching your target heart rate." (The rate is computed by subtracting your age from the number 220. Sixty-five percent of the resulting figure is your target rate per minute, which you should maintain for at least 20 minutes.)

There seems to be some doubt as to whether the Rotation Diet actually increases the metabolic rate as Dr. Katahn claims. While some of the experts contacted felt the 600- and 900-calorie rotations would probably decrease metabolic rate, others said the calorie increases to 1,200 and 1,800 in the ensuing rotations may indeed prevent a slowdown. Plus, exercise is a scientifically proven means of stimulating the metabolic rate, and the Rotation Diet insists on brisk physical activity. As one expert says, "There's no data that I know of to support his claim, but there's none to discredit it, either."

As for the vacation, "It sounds like a psychological trick designed to prime you from the beginning, to give you hope that there's light at the end of the tunnel if you just hold on through those first three hungry weeks," says William Bennett, M.D., a Harvard Medical School researcher who has studied eating disorders and diets and is coauthor of *The Dieter's Dilemma.* "I would guess the majority of the people will get off the diet at that point, however."

Says Dr. Harmatz, "If someone is overweight, you can't give them free rein over any type of food. People who overeat may do so in response to emotional needs, such as nervousness or depression. If you don't get to the root of the problem and solve it from that end, they'll just eat more and more of the so-called safe foods, until one day the safe foods don't satisfy anymore and they binge on high-calorie foods."

Needed: More Attention to Eating Behavior

The experts say the rotation plan, like so many other diets, is a Band-Aid treatment for a very complex problem. "These diets don't address the behavioral aspects of food consumption or the changes in life-style that are needed to achieve successful long-term weight control, instead of just temporary weight loss," Dr. Harmatz says. "Diets like the Rotation Diet give you a strict list of foods that are boring, especially when you think about them in terms of long periods. For any diet plan to work it has to be a commitment for extended periods. It's not a matter of losing 10 or 20 pounds and returning to old eating habits. If you do, the research shows you'll gain the weight right back—and maybe a few pounds more."

The diet made national news when cities, towns and neighborhoods from Colorado to Tennessee jumped on the rotation bandwagon and set mass weight-loss goals. Supermarket chains have also put foods for the Rotation Diet menus on sale and helped instill local weight-loss fervor. "The diet has gotten a lot of community support, and people get that initial boost of confidence and determination when they're in the grocery stores where the diets are being publicized," says psychologist Don Powell, Ph.D., executive director of the American Institute for Preventive Medicine in Southfield, Michigan. "But when they get home, they're faced with the same old urges to eat, and there's nothing to change those behavior patterns that lead to overeating. Their confidence succumbs to temptation."

So is there such a thing as an ideal weight-loss plan?

"It's not a matter of opening a book," says Musgrave. "If someone is serious about losing weight, they should look at the diets available, modify them to suit individual life-styles, and don't just accept them as is because that may not work."

According to Anderson, self-realization is the means to success. "Dieters need to discover for themselves what's causing their downfall. Do they eat because they're depressed, or are they habitual munchers who can't sit in front of the television without snacking? A lot of people don't think about how or why they gain weight. But once they're able to say, 'Oh yeah, that's why I'm eating so much,' we've found that they're more willing to modify their behavior and life-style so they can stick to a weight-loss plan. You have to take the responsibility and not rely on a prepackaged diet in a book that worked for someone else."

Once you've found your culinary Achilles' heel, making changes in eating and cooking habits—baking instead of cooking with fat and taking smaller portions on your plate, for instance—is a major step. "Choose a variety of foods to make eating as interesting as possible, because boredom kills a lot of diets," says Musgrave.

"Drastic Changes Rarely Work"

"Drastic changes rarely work, so make them gradually," she adds. "Few people can go from a candy bar one day to a stalk of celery the next. It may take two to three weeks to get down to 1,200 calories a day, but that's all right because you'll be slowly making changes that can be easily integrated into your life-style with little stress."

Dr. Harmatz also favors a temperate approach. "It's best to cut back just enough so there's a calorie loss without disrupting the normal life-style all at once.

"Take people who want to lose 10 or 15 pounds, for example. They don't need a drastic plan, just a diet that's subtly deficient in calories. If you eliminate 100 calories a day, eat a few less slices of bread or one less handful of peanuts and exercise more, in a year's time you've lost about 10 pounds. The problem is that most people don't want to wait a year."

Exercise, as Dr. Katahn stresses throughout his book, is crucial to weight loss and control. Says Dr. Bennett, "Of the things that we can manipulate to make us lose weight, we tend to underestimate the impact of exercise. If people would just find some type of aerobic activity that they enjoy and do it each day for at least 25 minutes or so, they'll do more for themselves in the long term than any diet could ever hope to do."

29 Little Ways to Lose a Lot of Weight

If Aladdin's lamp found its way into your hands, would you include weight loss on your list of three wishes? Do you feel nothing short of a miracle could make your unwanted pounds disappear?

The rub with losing weight is that we're usually better at wishing for slimness than attaining it. And sometimes we even try too hard, going on a rigid reducing regimen that eventually leaves our resolve limp as a rag. Here's another suggestion, with a lot less potential for backfiring: Take it easy.

"Your extra weight is the final result of many small behavioral acts, things like eating between meals or driving to places only two blocks away," explains Kelly Brownell, Ph.D., associate professor in the Department of Psychiatry at the University of Pennsylvania School of Medicine and co-director of the Obesity Research Clinic in Philadelphia. "So you can lose weight by making many small, clever changes—in diet, exercise and attitude."

For slow but sure weight loss, draft into your daily habits 10, 15 or more of the following little ways to lose weight. They're little because by themselves they probably won't make much difference. But together they can change your behavior just enough to get you eating better, moving more—losing more!

1.   Go grocery shopping on a full stomach. Nacho chips, dough-nuts and other tempters won't have half the allure they would if you hunted through those aisles hungry.

2.   Shop from a list of necessities. Allow yourself only one pur-chase that wasn't preplanned.

3.   Take only a limited amount of money when you shop. As an extra reinforcement against buying high-calorie foods, limit the amount you can spend.

4.   Invite your spouse or housemate into the kitchen. When you're preparing meals and cleaning up, a friend on the scene will help to keep you from sampling as you go.

5.   Don't eat foods out of their original containers. You may think you're having "just a tad," but you'll probably con-sume more than if you had dished out the food in a meas-ured portion. Better yet, don't bring your "weakness food" into the house in the first place. Present yourself with the hassle of going to the store for single servings if you can't fight off a craving. This way you'll either get some exercise (especially if you walk to the store), or you'll decide the snack isn't worth the bother after all.

6.   Eat only at scheduled times in scheduled places. A regimen helps you avoid unstructured eating.

7.   Use good plate psychology. Don't use place settings with intense colors such as violet, lime green, bright yellow or bright blue; they're thought to stimulate the appetite. The same goes for primitive-looking pewter and wooden plates. Instead, appease your appetite with elegant place settings in darker colors. Choose plates with broad decorative borders and a slightly "bowled" design. You can fit less food in them.

8.   Have someone else serve you, and ask for smaller portions.

9.   Police your eating speed. Put your fork down between bites. The slower you eat, the faster you'll feel full.

10. Establish a time-out routine. Halfway through your meals,

take a break. One trick: Put a large pot of water on the stove when you sit down to eat. When it boils (in about 10 or 15 minutes), get up and make a pot of herbal tea. When you go back to the table, you probably won't feel like eating much more.

11. Chew each bite of food at least ten times. This helps you really taste the food and makes you eat more slowly.

12. Don't eat everything on your plate. Make it a habit to always leave a little food, unless you're having steamed vegetables and fish, or an equally good-for-you meal.

13. Leave the table as soon as you're finished eating. Don't linger over the last bites.

14. Remove food stashed in inappropriate places. Get the candy bars out of your desk drawer and remove the nut bowl from the coffee table.

15. Use whipped or softened butter or margarine. You'll spread the flavor around using a lot less than if it was hard and you had to scrape it on.

16. Share desserts if skipping them is unthinkable.

17. Downscale your brand of ice cream. If it'll be a cold day in Key West before your freezer doesn't have a carton of this confection waiting for you, buy the least expensive or a reduced-fat brand. Your intake of fat and calories will be considerably lower than if you ate the gourmet kind.

18. Don't skip meals. You'll only overeat later.

19. Do more "fidgeting." For those of us who habitually squirm, toe tap or finger drum, it has been found in one study that fidgeting burns up to 800 calories a day in some people. That's the equivalent of jogging several miles.

   The problem, according to Eric Ravussin, Ph.D., visiting scientist with the National Institutes of Health and one of the study's researchers, is that "you really can't make your body have more spontaneous activity like fidgeting if you don't already do it. You can, however, decide to make your body work more whenever possible to burn extra calories.

   "Try doing things like getting up to switch TV channels

by hand instead of by remote control," he advises, "or putting frequently used books on higher shelves so you have to reach."

20. Swear off elevators and escalators. Take the stairs instead.

21. Fire the maid and do your own housework. Depending on your body weight, studies show you can burn 195 to 305 calories for each hour you spend washing windows, mopping floors and doing other tasks.

22. De-automate your housework and make your body work harder. Wash dishes, mix batters and open cans by hand, hang your wash on the line instead of using a dryer.

23. Exercise during television commercials. Those three-minute spurts will keep you out of the kitchen.

24. Go dancing, miniature golfing, bowling. If you normally sit around and play bridge or watch television, do anything active instead. The most calories you can burn in an hour playing cards is 95, but waltzing can whisk away 195 to 305 for every hour on the floor, and an hour of square dancing can stomp away 330 to 510 calories.

25. When you go out, drink no-calorie sparkling waters as a substitute for alcoholic beverages.

26. Get rid of those degrading signs and pictures on your refrigerator. Don't use images of 300-pound women in bikinis or pink pigs on beach blankets to shame you into not eating. Your willpower will be stronger from encouragement, not belittlement.

27. Hold a conference. Explain your weight-loss wish to family, friends or doughnut-bearing co-workers. Ask them to understand if you turn down their dinners or candy.

28. Learn that it's okay to say "No, thank you" when other people offer you food.

29. Set a realistic goal for yourself. "Take it one day at a time and don't punish yourself for slipping," says Suzann Johnson, nutritionist with Weight Watchers International, Inc. "You'll be more successful if you remember to be your own best friend."

C H A P T E R
E L E V E N

Fat-Removal Surgery: The Inside Story

Surgeon: First I'm going to put you to sleep. Then I'm going to make some tiny incisions here on your waist and each of your thighs and insert this suction tube and then switch on the suction and . . .

Patient: Will this hurt?

Surgeon: You won't feel a thing. I'll suck out all that ugly fat, just drain away your "saddlebags" and vacuum off those "love handles" forever. And when you wake up, you'll be down to a size 7 and won't have any scars or bruises or anything. You'll have to get rid of those size 13 dresses and buy some skintight jeans to show off the beautiful new you. You'll want to wear a bikini on the beach and you'll get whistled at a lot and . . .

Such a fantasy surely danced in the heads of hundreds when the news first broke about suction lipectomy, the latest fat-removing technique imported from France. And, apparently, the dream of instant svelte dies hard.

Practitioners of the art (mostly plastic surgeons and dermatologists) have been trying to curb some of the wishful thinking, but the procedure's image as a "magic bullet" against flab and sag persists. More than 4,000 Americans have submitted to the treatment, and more candidates are queuing up from coast to coast.

The operation is the newest technique in an old trend toward "fat surgery," the radical tactic in the war on flab. It follows the intestinal bypass, gastric bypass, gastroplasty and a long list of variations on them all.

Their proponents are the first to point out that the procedures are for the select few—the seriously obese or, in the case of suction lipectomy, those with well-entrenched clumps of fat here and there. But the appeal of the surgical operation is strong. Some people no doubt view fat surgery as a way around the brutal arithmetic of all weight gain: When calorie intake exceeds calorie expenditure, the result is fat, often just where you don't want it. For them, solving the caloric arithmetic is a long, hard road, and fat surgery is a waiting taxi.

Even with inflated expectations aside, the surgeon's answer to flab has always been overshadowed by looming questions. And perhaps the most compelling ones are those that come most readily to the layman's lips: Does the operation work, and is it safe?

Scooping Up Lipids

Darlene K., 33, of Andrews, North Carolina, wondered just that about lipectomy and then last year decided to give it a try. "I'm four feet, 11 inches tall and weighed only 100 pounds at the time of the operation," she says. "But I had saddlebag thighs and desperately wanted to get rid of them."

The surgeon anesthetized her from the waist down, using local anesthetic (general anesthetic is often used, too), gave her intravenous Valium and completed the procedure in half an hour. Two hours later she was hobbling about, and in five days she was back at work.

She had to wear a girdlelike bandage for a week, and her thighs hurt for four days. For a month they were sore and bruised, and for two months there was numbness in one of them. "I think it was worth the risk," she says. "My saddlebags are gone, and that's all that matters."

Donna C., 35, of Richmond, Virginia, got the saddlebag treatment, too, along with many of the same aftereffects. "The operation took two inches off each thigh," she says. "I wouldn't say that the results are cosmetically perfect, but I'm never going to have Betty Grable legs anyway. There's some slight waviness in the skin, which they say will eventually smooth out."

The Limits of "Magic"

So it seems that sucking away fat is trickier than it looks, as novice practitioners have found out. The surgeon first must make a ½-inch incision in the skin at the least noticeable corner of the lipectomy site. Then he has to insert into the opening a foot-long metal tube (a cannula) about the thickness of a pencil, which is connected by plastic tubing to a suction pump. He moves the cannula up and back through the fatty deposits, between muscle below and skin above, slowly drawing out the fat.

"This seemingly simple procedure is not simple at all," says Joseph Agris, M.D., Houston plastic surgeon and coauthor of *Suction-Assisted Lipectomy Clinical Atlas.* "The surgeon has to make sure that he maneuvers the instrument in the proper plane. He must have good eye/finger coordination to avoid severing blood vessels and nerves. And he has to remove just the right amount of fat from all areas to ensure a symmetrical appearance. If he suctions away too much at any given spot, he risks creating a hollow that is impossible to fill and may cause an unsightly indentation in the skin."

It's this apparent simplicity that worries plastic surgeons most. They fear that it might entice a few money-minded but untrained colleagues to wield the cannula on patients who could get along fine with no fat removal at all.

That fear was voiced by none other than the American Society of Plastic and Reconstructive Surgeons (ASPRS). A report from the society that cautiously endorsed the suction treatment stated, "This procedure could be overutilized by quasi practitioners or untrained physicians who apply it to minimal or inappropriate deformities for maximum reimbursement, thereby generating significant criticism."

Such a blunt warning doesn't come a moment too soon, for some plastic surgeons privately admit that there are some medical professionals now performing suction operations without the requisite skills.

Not the least of said skills is careful patient screening. According to the ASPRS, suction lipectomy is *not* just for anybody with a weight problem, and any worthy practitioner will make that clear to every candidate that comes along.

"The procedure is not for weight control and certainly not for obesity," says Samuel J. Stegman, M.D., associate clinical professor of dermatology at the University of California, San Francisco. "It's for men and women close to their ideal weight, with good skin elasticity, who want to shed specific deposits of bulging fat (such as on the buttocks, thighs, chin and abdomen) that diet and exercise can't eliminate."

Most practitioners agree with these stipulations and would even tack on age limitations. Some use the suction procedure only on patients 45 and younger. Others set the maximum age at 35. After all, age is a reliable indicator of the suppleness of skin, a factor that could influence whether the treated area looks like normal human flesh or like a fallen soufflé.

"The candidate must have excellent skin tone," Dr. Agris says. "When the fat is suctioned away, the skin has to shrink to the body's new contours."

And that's also a good reason for the caveat against using suction lipectomy to help somebody drop 20 pounds. The skin's ability to contract limits the amount of fat that can be taken from any one area at a time. It's theorized that if too much fat is suctioned off the back of the skin, it may lead to ripples.

Or worse. Too much fat removal, and the patient could go into fluid-loss shock. As the fat tissue is sucked out, the fluids trickle into the void and get drawn out, too. It's little wonder that the better practitioners set limits on the amount of fat they'll remove in any single operation: three pounds or less per session.

Gauging the Gamble

But sometimes even with the right patient and the right surgeon, things can go wrong. This procedure has its risks like any other kind of surgery. Most people who have the operation are generally satisfied with the results and have few complications, but some wish they had let well enough alone.

"There are some complications that worry me more than others," says Kelman Cohen, M.D., chairman of plastic surgery at the Medical College of Virginia in Richmond. "They are blood loss, fluid loss and hematoma [hemorrhage under the skin]. And, of course, the likelihood of these problems is greatest among unqualified practitioners." This is why Dr. Cohen feels this procedure is best done by plastic surgeons.

The ASPRS worries about complications, too. Their report on suction lipectomy mentions the possibility of skin dimpling (what they call a "cottage cheese" skin texture), fluid retention, pain, asymmetry in fat removal, waviness in the skin, pigmentation problems, scarring, skin sloughing (peeling away) and permanent numbness.

The worst possibility, however, is not on the list: perforation of the abdomen. Plastic surgeons say that it would be easy for an untrained and unhandy practitioner to push the cannula right through the abdominal wall.

Perhaps the most unsettling fact about the procedure is that it's so new that there's little precise data on the probability of complications. Plastic surgeons say the risks are within acceptable limits, but the unknown nag nonetheless.

There are even questions about the permanence of the postoperative results. After fat is suctioned off, can it eventually come back? Can remaining fat cells enlarge and thus neutralize the surgeon's efforts? Will fat surrounding the suctioned area sooner or later crowd into the artificial gap? Plenty of practitioners would love to know. And since a suction lipectomy costs $300 to $4,000 (depending on the areas suctioned), many candidates would probably like to find out, too.

Bypassing Willpower

We know far more, however, about the forerunner of all fat surgery—the intestinal (jejunoileal) bypass. For over three decades surgeons have used it as a last-resort cure for people who are "morbidly obese"—those weighing more than 100 pounds over their ideal weight. Thousands have undergone the operation, and thousands have been followed up months or even years later for postoperative evaluation.

The procedure's claim to fame is that it forces weight loss upon the patient by short-circuiting the anatomy. The surgeon accomplishes the feat by coupling the beginning of the small intestine to its end (a few inches before the colon), bypassing about 20 feet of its length. The excised portion becomes anatomical excess baggage. The result is that food can't be fully digested, and huge bundles of calories get expelled instead of absorbed. For most bypass patients, this means rapid loss of extra pounds.

It can also mean disaster. Several reports have condemned the operation because it creates more problems than it solves. They document a startling array of possible complications—liver disease, bone disease, kidney stones, protein malabsorption, infection, gallstones, inflammation of the intestines, nutrient deficiency, severe diarrhea, vomiting, even arthritis.

More to the point, in some cases the intestinal bypass has proved lethal. Up to 6 percent of patients die on the operating table, and the overall mortality rate may be much higher—mostly due to liver deterioration. At least 91 people have died from postoperative liver disease.

In an indictment of the intestinal bypass, a group of surgeons at the University of Kentucky Medical Center at Lexington declared, "It is our contention that a 50 percent morbidity [complication] rate and roughly a 10 percent mortality following jejunoileal bypass are sufficient reason to abandon it as an appropriate operation for the morbidly obese."

Getting around the Stomach

It's no wonder then that most obesity surgeons have switched to the less troublesome gastric procedures, what some people call stomach stapling. The operations—for desperately obese people only—are designed to ensure drastic weight loss by performing surgical sleight-of-hand on the patient's stomach and appetite.

The trick involves partitioning the stomach with steel staples so that there's a small pouch near the top, the first stop for food on its way to digestion. In the surgical variation called gastric bypass, an opening is created in the side of the pouch, and a section of small intestine is connected to it to carry food through the lower tract. The lower part of the stomach becomes a useless hollow. In a version called gastroplasty, a small passage is formed between the pouch and the much larger lower stomach. Food enters the pouch, then trickles slowly through the passage and down to the lower stomach and bowel. Regardless of the gastric replumbing, the result is the same: The pouch prevents a large food intake and fools the patient into believing that a few bites are quite enough.

The deception works most of the time. In a study of 167 people who had gastric surgery, Lloyd D. MacLean, M.D. a Quebec surgeon, and his colleagues report that 60 percent of the patients lost at least one-quarter of their preoperative weight. Twenty-six percent of them, however, were judged to have "unsatisfactory" weight loss.

Unfortunately, many of the 167 paid dearly for the lost pounds. "Malnutrition developed in a significant number of the patients," says Dr. MacLean. "The effect was mostly due to their reduced dietary intake."

Because of this complication, as well as inadequate weight loss and obstructed intestines, 71 of the operations had to be redone.

Other reports detail a wide range of complications for gastric bypass—from infection to hair loss to blood clots in the lungs—and say that more than 30 percent of patients experience them. They give

Body Sculpting
without the Surgeon

Is it possible to shed specific lumps of body fat—to "body sculpt"—without surgery? Experts say yes—sort of.

"It's probably not feasible to spot-reduce deposits of fat," says Ronald Mackenzie, M.D., medical director of the National Athletic Health Institute in Inglewood, California. "But it is possible to achieve an equivalent result. Through exercise you can strengthen muscles and improve posture so fat areas appear much less noticeable. And by a combination of diet and exercise you can reduce total body fat and thus enhance your overall appearance.

"All this is especially true of the abdominal area, where increasing muscle tone often means greatly enhancing a slimmed-down look."

gastroplasty better marks, but point to bone loss, stretching of the stomach pouch and bowel obstruction as the more serious after-surgery problems. And neither type of operation can claim a long-term mortality rate any lower than 1 percent.

"Gastric stapling hasn't stood the test of time," says William E. Straw, M.D., of the Palo Alto Medical Foundation in California. "I worry that the procedure, like the intestinal bypass, may eventually prove medically unsound. Such operations may be warranted for some severely obese people whose weight is life-threatening. But in my work with the morbidly obese, I've found safer — but perhaps less glamorous — alternatives: They're called diet and exercise."